FOOD
AND NUTRITION
FOR YOU

Anne Barnett

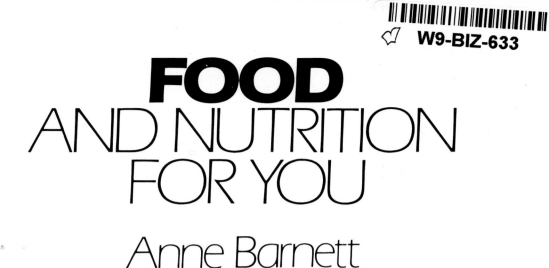

FOOD
AND NUTRITION
FOR YOU

Anne Barnett

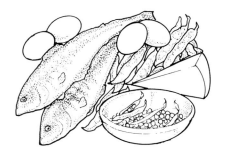

Hutchinson

London   Melbourne   Sydney   Auckland   Johannesburg

Hutchinson Education

An imprint of the Century Hutchinson Publishing Group
62–65 Chandos Place, London WC2N 4NW

Century Hutchinson Australia Pty Ltd
PO Box 496, 16–22 Church Street, Hawthorn, Victoria 3122,
Australia

Century Hutchinson New Zealand Ltd
PO Box 40–086, Glenfield, Auckland 10, New Zealand

Century Hutchinson South Africa (Pty) Ltd
PO Box 337, Bergvlei 2012, South Africa

First published 1985
Reprinted 1985, 1986, 1987

British Library Cataloguing in Publication Data

Barnett, Anne
    Food and nutrition for you.
    1. Nutrition
    I. Title
613.2   TX 354

ISBN 0 09 159311 5

Acknowledgements

Thanks are due to the following for permission to reproduce
photographs: Banbury Guardian p.38; Barnaby's Picture
Library pp.69, 70, 81, 90, 99, 101, 110, 119; Birds Eye Wall's
Ltd pp.102, 111; Anthony Blake pp.4, 23, 26, 46, 69, 70, 71, 81,
99; The British Arkady Co. Ltd p.9; British Gas pp.86, 119;
British Meat pp.49, 52; J. Allan Cash Ltd pp.12, 23, 29, 30, 32,
34, 44, 66, 97; Denby Tableware Ltd p.92; Eggs Information
Bureau pp.56, 58; English Country Cheese Council pp.63, 97;
The Flour Advisory Bureau pp.79, 82; Milk Marketing Board
pp.61, 62; Philips Electronics pp.86, 87, 103; The Prestige
Group PLC pp.75, 89, 90; J Sainsbury PLC pp.32, 33; Sea Fish
Industry Authority p.54; Tesco Stores Ltd pp.83, 97, 101, 119;
T. I. Tower Housewares Ltd p.91.

Tables on pages 12 and 42 are reproduced by permission of
the Controller of Her Majesty's Stationery Office.

Examination questions are reproduced by permission of the
following examination boards: Associated Lancashire
Schools Examining Board; East Midlands Regional
Examinations Board; Joint Matriculation Board; London
Regional Examinations Board; Northern Examining
Association; The South-East Regional Examinations Board;
Southern Regional Examination Board; University of
Cambridge Local Examinations Syndicate; Welsh Joint
Education Committee.

Designed and illustrated by
The Pen and Ink Book Co. Ltd

Cartoons by Dave Parkin
Illustrations of food by Ahmet

Phototypeset in 11 on 13pt Gill Light by
The Pen and Ink Book Co Ltd

Printed and bound in Great Britain by
Butler & Tanner Ltd.

Contents

1 Introducing food

1.1	Introduction	4
1.2	Nutrients	5
1.3	Proteins	7
1.4	Starches and sugars (carbohydrates)	10
1.5	Fats and oils (lipids)	11
1.6	Energy	12
1.7	Vitamins	14
1.8	Minerals	18
Recap 1		22

2 Planning and balancing meals

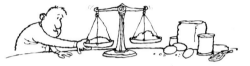

2.1	A balanced diet	23
2.2	Special needs	24
2.3	Saving fuel	25
2.4	Meal patterns	26
2.5	Breakfast	27
2.6	Midday meal	28
2.7	The main meal of the day	30
2.8	Shops and shopping	31
Recap 2		35

3 Diets and health

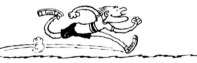

3.1	Vegetarians	36
3.2	Some ethnic groups	37
3.3	Elderly people	38
3.4	People living alone	39
3.5	People on a small budget	40
3.6	People recovering from an illness	41
3.7	Over-eating	42
3.8	Too much sugar	44
3.9	Heart disease	45
3.10	Dietary fibre and bowel disease	46
Recap 3		47

4 The food we eat

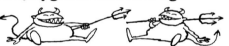

4.1	Meat	48
4.2	Fish	53
4.3	Eggs	56
4.4	Milk	60
4.5	Cheese	63
4.6	Fruit	65
4.7	Vegetables	67
4.8	Cereals	69
Recap 4		73

5 Cooking

5.1	Food and cooking	74
5.2	Raising agents	78
5.3	Food and heat	84
5.4	Cookers and ovens	86
5.5	Cooking materials	90
Recap 5		93

6 Food, hygiene and storage

6.1	Food and bacteria	94
6.2	Food and spoilage	97
6.3	Nutrition and preserved food	99
6.4	Kitchen hygiene	101
6.5	Waste disposal	105
Recap 6		107

7 Food and technology

7.1	Food additives	108
7.2	Convenience foods	110
Recap 7		113

Revision	114
Examinations	115
Exam questions	116
Careers	119
Index	120

1 Introducing food

1.1 Introduction

This book is about food. Most of us enjoy thinking about food and eating it. But have you ever thought about why we eat food, apart from the enjoyment?

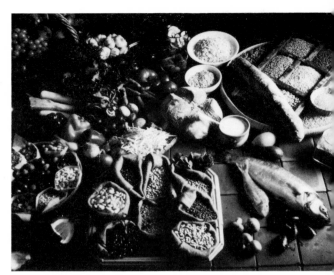

Food is enjoyable

What does food do?

Food does the following jobs:

1 It builds and repairs the body.
2 It supplies enough energy for a person to work, play and keep warm and to keep the body 'ticking over' when it is resting.
3 It protects the body from disease and helps it to use food efficiently. This is called **regulating your body processes**.

To live life to the full we must be fit and energetic and enjoy living. Many things help to make us feel like this. The most important is eating the right foods for health and enjoyment. This unit is about which foods are needed for our own 'recipe' for good health.

   Get into the habit of making a link between **food eaten** and **activities**. You will then find it easy to plan food for yourself and others. Think of the foods you eat as ingredients for a product, energy, which you use for activities and keeping healthy. Foods eaten and energy are like scales because they should balance.

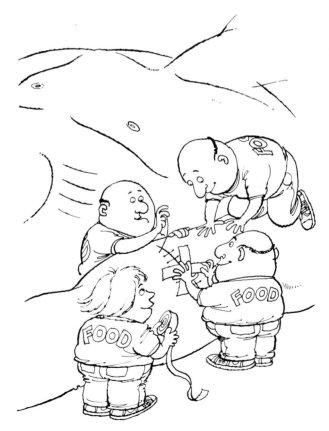

Things to do

1 *Make a list of the foods you have eaten already today. Add the foods you are likely to eat later.*

2 *Make another list of the activities you have carried out. For example: got up, dressed, walked to school.*

3 *Do you think your two lists balance? Later you will learn how to do this accurately.*

4

1.2 Nutrients

Food can be divided into a number of parts which do different jobs in the body. These parts are called nutrients. All food contains nutrients, but hardly any food contains them all. This means that we need to eat a variety of foods to get all the nutrients we need for good health.

The nutrients

Your recipe for good health should contain all of the following ingredients:

1 **Proteins** — these are used for body-building and repair. They are the 'building blocks' of the body.
2 **Starches and sugars (carbohydrates)** — these are used for energy. Think of them as the 'fuel' of your body.
3 **Fats and oils (lipids)** — these are also used for energy and warmth.
4 **Vitamins and mineral salts** — each different vitamin and mineral salt does several different jobs in your body. They help your body to make good use of the other nutrients and protect itself from disease.
5 **Water** — this is the essential liquid in which every body process takes place. A shortage of water is dangerous to health.
6 **Dietary fibre** — this is sometimes called **roughage**. Dietary fibre is an indigestible material which is not absorbed by the body. It helps the body to dispose of waste material efficiently.

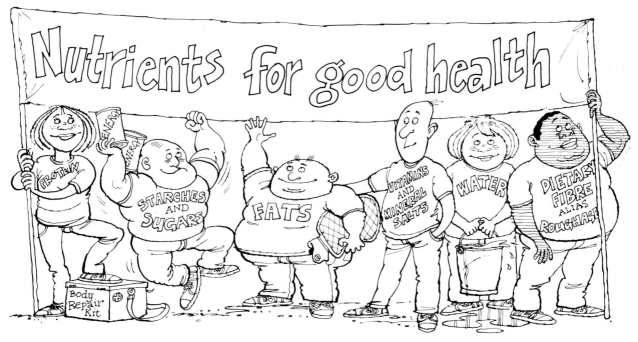

Nutrients from food

To have good health we need to choose food wisely. Unfortunately we can't just go out and buy nutrients because shops don't sell them. Instead, we need to know the **food sources** of the nutrients. We need to discover the nutritive value of the foods we can buy. This study of foods is called **nutrition**.

Some facts about nutrients

Most foods contain more than one nutrient. Some foods contain a large amount of one nutrient and small amounts of others. Because of this they are used as a main food source of the nutrient they contain a large amount of. For example, meat and fish both contain many nutrients, but the one they contain most of is high value protein so they are both used as main food sources of protein.

Sometimes, a food can be a main food source of a nutrient just because a lot of the food is eaten, rather than because the food has a lot of the nutrient in it. Potatoes are a good example of this. Potatoes do not contain a large amount of vitamin C, but because they are eaten in most main meals in the UK, the amount of vitamin C supplied by them is high in most people's diet.

Things to do

1 *Design a poster about nutrients. Call your poster 'The recipe for good health'. Put it up in your home economics room.*

2 *Find out about food sources of nutrients. See if you can find two food sources for each nutrient in the recipe for good health.*

1.3 Proteins

Protein is the nutrient used for body-building and repair.

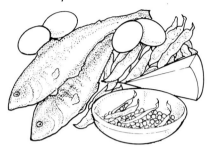

The two types of protein

Proteins are made up of different parts called **amino acids**. Human body flesh is made up of proteins which must contain certain of these amino acids called **essential** amino acids. Animal sources of protein contain more of these essential amino acids than vegetable sources. This is why meat, fish, cheese, eggs and milk are of higher biological value.

The main food sources of protein

We get protein from two main types of food:

1 Animal sources — this is **protein of higher biological value (HBV)** or **high value protein**. Examples of foods containing this are meat, fish, cheese, eggs and milk.

2 Vegetable sources — this is **protein of lower biological value (LBV)** or **low value protein**. Food examples of this are peas, beans, lentils, nuts and cereals. (Soya beans are an exception as although they are a vegetable source they contain protein of HBV. See page 9 for more about this.)

Both of these sources of protein are important.

Proteins from vegetable sources do not contain all the essential amino acids. This means that by themselves they cannot supply all the protein the body needs to build and repair tissues. This is why protein from vegetable sources is of lower biological value. However, a combination of foods supplying lower biological value protein, e.g. beans on toast, can mean that the amino acid which is missing in one of the foods is supplied by the other.

Some facts about proteins

Fact	Using the fact
1 The body cannot store protein.	We need to eat food supplying protein every day. Different people need different amounts. For example, a girl aged between 12 and 15 needs between 44 and 58 grams of protein each day.
2 If too much protein is eaten one day it cannot be carried over to the next. The body will turn it into energy.	It is bad planning to have too much protein one day and none the next. Protein foods are dearer sources of energy than starches and sugars.
3 Proteins from animal sources and proteins from vegetable sources are complementary.	Meals should be planned to include foods from both sources. As vegetables are usually cheaper to buy than foods from animal sources, this is a good thing to do to help the household budget.
4 Lower biological value protein is not inferior to higher biological value protein.	Two or more lower biological value protein foods can be used together in the same dish or meal. In this way one protein food supplies the amino acids which the other protein food may lack.

Balancing your proteins

Nutritionally it is a good idea to serve some food containing protein from animal sources with some food containing protein from vegetable sources in the same meal. Having food that supplies a mixture of protein from vegetable and cereal sources together is also a good idea. This means that each type of protein can make up for what the other lacks. When proteins are used like this we say that they **complement** or **supplement** each other. Balancing your proteins like this also saves you money because vegetables and cereals are cheaper than foods from animal sources.

Some examples of meals with balanced proteins are:

Sausage and baked beans
Bread and cheese
Spaghetti bolognaise
Mixed vegetable cobbler
Onion and bean quiche
Beans on toast
Lentil soup and bread rolls

Getting enough protein

How do we know how much protein is in different foods? The following provides us with 12 g of protein:

Protein of higher biological value

75 g liver
75 g coley or cod
75 g beef
50 g cheese
100 g eggs — (How many eggs is this? To find the weight of the edible portion of each egg, subtract the weight of the shell from the weight of the whole egg.)
500ml milk

Protein of lower biological value

6 slices white bread
200 g baked beans — (How many tins is this? Read the label to see how much is in each tin.)
42 g peanuts
600 g potatoes

Most people probably have more than enough protein. Some doctors think that we could be perfectly healthy with less. The table shows the amount of protein recommended per day for some groups of people. These recommendations are only a guide though, because our needs vary.

Type of person	Recommended amount of protein per day (g)	Minimum amount of protein per day (g)
Children 7-8 yrs	53	30
Boys 15-17 yrs	75	50
Girls 15-17 yrs	58	40
Men 18-34 yrs		
Sedentary	68	45
Very active	90	45
Women 18-34 yrs		
Most occupations	55	38
Pregnant	60	44
Lactating	68	55

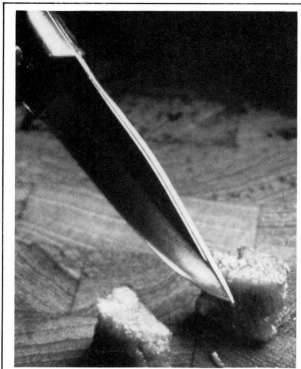

Cutting TVP

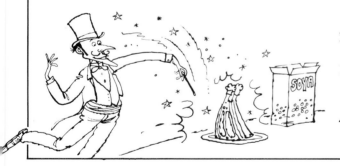

Making meat from a vegetable

Soya beans contain protein of higher biological value just like meat. But they are a much cheaper source than meat. Food manufacturers have found ways of making soya beans look and taste like meat. They make the beans into **textured vegetable protein (TVP)**.

Protein from soya beans is spun into fibres and treated in different ways to make it look like beef, pork or chicken. It can be bought as joints, chops, chunks or mince. It also has other nutrients added to it to make it more nutritious. This is called **fortification**. TVP is fortified with iron and vitamins from the B group to make it nutritionally as valuable as meat.

Why bother to make TVP?

TVP has many advantages:

1. It is cheaper to provide a portion of, for example, bolognaise sauce made from TVP, than it is to provide a portion made from fresh meat.
2. TVP can be used to make fresh meat go further. This is called **extending**.
3. TVP is easy to store. It is bought dried in a packet or in a sauce in a can and it keeps well for a long time.
4. TVP is useful to have as a stand by in emergencies.

Things to do

1. *Think of some more examples of meals with a balanced supply of proteins.*

2. *Compare the cost of making a beefburger containing*
   a *100 g fresh mince and*
   b *50 g fresh mince and 50 g (after soaking) of TVP beef mince.*

3. *Prepare beefburgers using the ingredients in*

   2a and b and compare the difference in
   a *taste,*   d *cooking time,*
   b *texture,*   e *appearance.*
   c *ease of mixing,*

4. *Look for the number of different ways in which TVP is offered for sale. Look especially at the list of ingredients on ready-made pies, sausages, casseroles and so on.*

1.4 Starches and sugars (carbohydrates)

*All food has energy value. Some foods have higher energy value than other foods. These foods are called **high energy foods**. Examples of high energy foods are starches and sugars. These are often called **carbohydrates**.*

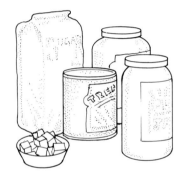

Sugars

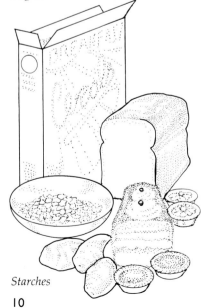

Starches

Sugars

These include all the obviously sweet things such as granulated, castor and icing sugar, treacle, honey and jam. Sugar has a high energy value but supplies no other nutrient. This is why it is sometimes called an **empty calorie food**. Sugary foods are fairly cheap to buy and are 'instant' to use.

Starches

Starch is found in foods like bread, cereals and potatoes. It is also found in floury, filling foods like pastries and cakes. Most of the foods which contain starch also contain other nutrients. For example, potatoes also supply vitamin C and bread supplies protein and calcium.

How much energy-giving food do we need?

The amount of energy-giving food which you eat must balance with the amount of energy your body needs for movement and activities. If you eat too much energy-giving food (particularly sugar) and you do not turn it into energy by working or exercise then your body will change the food into fat and store it away under your skin. This is how people put on weight and become fat (**obese**). Unfortunately, it is very easy to eat too much sweet food because it is easy and cheap to buy and many people find it comforting. (Have you ever bought a bag of sweets to cheer yourself up?)

Which foods supply the most energy?

The table below shows the percentage of energy provided by some foods. Remember that sugar is all energy.

Food	%	Food	%
Sugar	100	Potatoes	20
Jam and biscuits	70	Fruit, peas, beans	10
Bread	55	Green vegetables	4
Chocolate	55		

Things to do

1   *Explain why people can become fat if they eat too much.*

2   *Unjumble the following to find foods which contain sugars or starches:*

stopotae	*ronfackles*	*lodegn spryu*
lamadream	*dreab*	*ffoete*

1.5 Fats and oil (lipids)

*Fats and oils are also high energy foods. They are sometimes called **lipids**.*

Sources of fats

There are two kinds of fats found in food:

1 **Visible fats** (fats which you can see) as in butter, lard, margarine, cream and fatty meat.
2 **Invisible fats** (fats which are in the food but cannot be seen) as in cakes, biscuits, pastry, ice cream, sausages, oily fish such as herring and food cooked in fat such as chips.

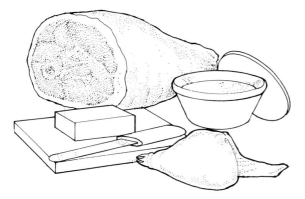

Visible fat food sources

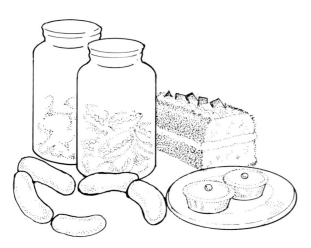

Invisible fat food sources

Using fats for energy

Fat gives more energy per gram than sugar and starch. It is a **compact** source of energy. Because it is so concentrated, a lot of heat is produced when fats are used for energy. They give warmth as well as energy to the body.

Other reasons for using fats

Fats are made up of **fatty acids** and **glycerol**. Some of these fatty acids are needed for healthy skin and proper growth in children. These are called **essential** fatty acids.

Most of the essential fatty acids we need are found in the plant sources of fats and oils, such as peanuts, olives, sunflowers and coconuts. Some margarines and cooking oils are made from these sources.

Which foods contain the most fat?

The table below shows the percentage of fat in some foods:

Food	%
Cooking fats and oils	100
Butter and margarine	80
Cheddar cheese	30
Meat	25
Oily fish	15
Eggs	10
Bread	5
Milk	4

Things to do

1 *List as many foods as you can which contain fats.*

2 *Explain what is meant by 'essential' fatty acid.*

3 *Make a study of margarines and cooking oils in your local supermarket. How many different plant sources of fats and oils can you find?*

1.6 Energy

Why we need energy

Our bodies use food for energy rather like a car uses petrol. Every time we move we use energy. Even when our bodies are sleeping they need energy because our hearts are still beating and many other organs are working. All our body processes use up energy.

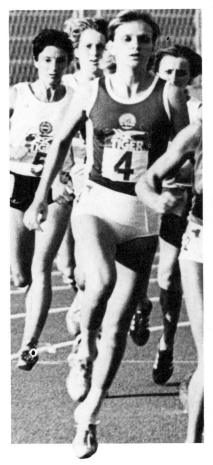

Where do we get energy from?

There are three main food sources of energy:

1. sugars and starches (carbohydrates),
2. fats and oils (lipids),
3. proteins which have not been used for body-building and repair.

How do we turn food into energy?

We get energy from food by **oxidizing** it. This is a process which happens when a substance reacts with oxygen. It is called **oxidation**. It is rather like burning things in air. But it happens much more slowly in our bodies and the energy does not just escape into the air. Instead, the energy is used for movement.

Oxidation works like this. Oxygen (in the air) is brought into our bodies through our lungs. It dissolves in our blood and is carried round in the blood stream. The substance in our bodies which reacts with this oxygen is called **glucose**. This is what we get when we digest sugars and starches. The glucose is also carried round in our bodies. This is what happens when the oxygen and glucose react:

oxygen + glucose → water, energy and carbon dioxide

Because we need energy all the time, this reaction never stops. The energy we produce allows us to move. The production of energy also makes heat so we can keep warm. The other products are water and carbon dioxide. We don't need these so we breathe them out through our lungs.

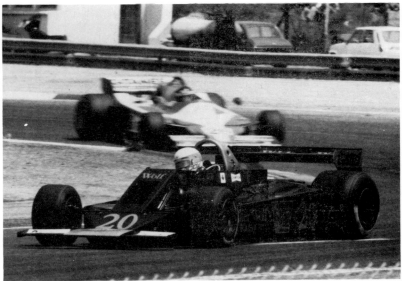

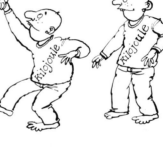

How can we measure the amount of energy in our food?

It is important to balance the amount of food we eat with the amount of energy we use. To make sure that the scales balance we just need to remember that energy can be measured just as temperature can be measured.

Energy supplied by food is measured in kilojoules (kJ). This is a metric unit. The old unit was the kilocalorie or Calorie with a capital C. As this is still sometimes used, it is useful to know how to convert kilocalories into kilojoules. Just remember:

4.2 kilojoules = 1 kilocalorie

or, easier still, a kilocalorie is roughly four times as big as a kilojoule.

Activities	Energy used kJ/min
Sleeping	4
Sitting	6
Standing	7
Washing	7
Dressing	7
Walking slowly	13
Walking quickly	21
Walking up and down stairs	38
Cycling	25
Dancing	25
Tennis	25
Cross-country running	35
Football	35
Swimming	35

Things to do

1   *Make a list of the foods you ate yesterday, and the rough amounts of each one. Try to calculate their energy value. The food tables in the* Manual of Nutrition *will help you to do this.*

2   *List the activities you carried out, including getting up, washing, getting dressed and watching television as well as running for the bus and playing games. Calculate how many kilojoules you used. Use the information in the box to help you and the table on page 43.*

3   *Compare the two calculations. Do they balance?*

1.7 **Vitamins**

Vitamins protect our bodies and regulate their functions. Part of their job is to ensure that the other nutrients do their work efficiently.

Some facts about vitamins

The table shows the main vitamins we need and the foods which contain them.

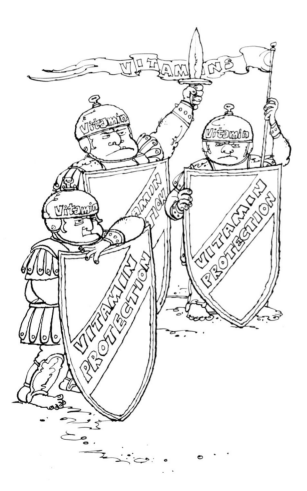

Vitamin	Food sources
Vitamin A (this can appear as **carotene** in yellow and red fruits and vegetables)	Fortified margarine, dairy products, milk, oil (particularly cod-liver oil and halibut-liver oil), carrots, green vegetables
Vitamin B Group B_1 Thiamin	Bread, flour, meat, potatoes, milk, fortified breakfast cereals
B_2 Riboflavin	Milk, meat (particularly liver), eggs, yeast extract
Nicotinic acid	Meat, bread, flour, fortified breakfast cereals, milk, liver, kidney, yeast extract
B_{12} Cobalamin	Produced in the intestines by bacteria, so it mainly comes from animal foods. Liver is the richest source
Folic acid	Offal, raw green leafy vegetables, pulses, bread, oranges, bananas
Vitamin C (sometimes called **ascorbic acid**)	Green vegetables, citrus fruits (lemons, oranges, limes), blackcurrants, rose-hip syrup
Vitamin D	Fortified margarine, fatty fish, eggs, butter, and the action of sunlight on the skin

Functions	Effects of shortage
Promotes good eyesight, healthy skin and linings of the body, normal growth.	Skin disorders, night blindness.
Helps to release energy from sugars and starches.	Lack of energy. Severe shortage causes **beri-beri**.
Helps to release energy from food, especially amino acids and fat. Promotes normal growth in children.	Severe shortage is rare, but when it does occur the lips, tongue and skin are affected.
Helps to release energy from food, especially carbohydrate. Essential for normal growth.	Nervous and digestive systems are affected. Severe shortage causes **pellagra**.
Helps the metabolism of amino acids and other body enzyme systems.	Special types of anaemia can occur where red blood cells become enlarged. Vegans are at risk because they do not eat any food from animals.
Helps B_{12} to divide cells.	Anaemia. Elderly people, pregnant women and premature infants could be at risk if there is a shortage in their diet.
Provides healthy connective tissues. Helps to rebuild new tissues and heal wounds.	Bleeding, particularly of the gums. Slow healing of wounds. Severe shortage causes **scurvy**.
Maintains the level of calcium in the blood to form strong bones and teeth.	**Rickets** in babies and young children. Bone softening (**osteomalacia**) in adults. Possible tooth decay.

Vitamin A

Vitamin A appears in fatty foods because it is **fat soluble**. This means it dissolves in fat.

Carotene, which is referred to in the table, can be changed into vitamin A in the body. The amount of carotene found in carrots and in dark green or yellow vegetables can be seen by their colour. The deeper the colour, the more carotene there is. The dark outer leaves of cabbage contain more carotene than the pale inner heart. The green grass which cows eat contains vitamin A. This is why dairy foods are such a rich source of the vitamin.

Vitamin A is stored in the liver. A well-fed adult will have a store which will last several months. Younger people may not have such a store so they should have a daily supply from the foods listed in the table. A particularly good source is margarine which is fortified with vitamin A by law.

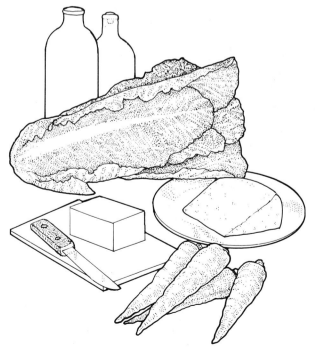

Vitamin D

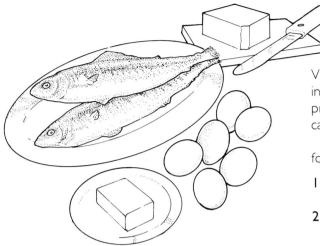

Vitamin D is another fat soluble vitamin. It is found in fatty foods. Sunlight is an important factor in the provision of vitamin D for most people. Our bodies can make vitamin D when sunlight falls on our skin.

Some people must have extra vitamin D from food. They are:

1 Children, pregnant women and lactating women (those breast feeding their babies).
2 People whose skin does not get much sunlight, such as the housebound or those who cover all their body with clothes.

Some foods are fortified with vitamin D by law, for example, margarine and some milk products (particularly dried milk for babies). There is no recommended daily supply except for the people mentioned above.

There is a link between vitamin D and the mineral calcium. Without a supply of vitamin D our bodies are unable to absorb calcium.

The B group vitamins

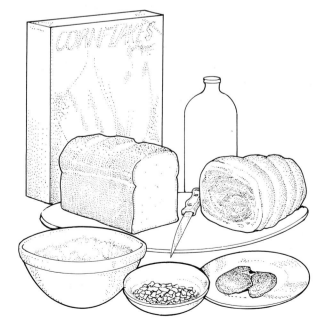

The main job of the B group vitamins is to help our bodies release energy from food. Look at the table of vitamins on pages 14 and 15. Check the names of the B group vitamins given there. They are **thiamin**, **riboflavin**, **nicotinic acid** (also called **niacin**), **cobalamin** and **folic acid**. Notice also that they tend to occur in the same foods.

The B group vitamins cannot be stored in the body for long because they are **water soluble**, they dissolve in water. This means that we need a daily supply of them. The amount we need depends on how much energy we use. A very energetic person requires more vitamin-B-rich food than a less energetic person.

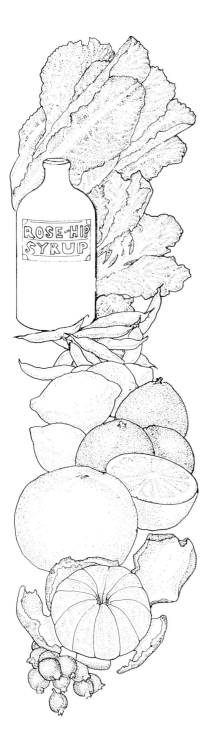

Vitamin C

Vitamin C is another water soluble vitamin. This means that care must be taken when preparing vitamin-C-rich foods because the vitamin can easily be lost. Vitamin C can dissolve in cooking water if the food is cooked for too long or in too much water.

The body cannot store vitamin C, so we need a daily supply. Young teenagers between the ages of 12 and 14 need at least 25 mg a day. If you remember that there is about 50 mg of vitamin C in an orange weighing 100 g, you can see an easy way of providing your daily supply.

Making the most of vitamin C in foods

Here are some ways of improving the vitamin C value of some foods which do not contain very much of the vitamin.

1   Soak dried fruit such as prunes or figs in orange or grapefruit juice and cook them in the juice.
2   Mix apples with tinned blackcurrants, blackcurrant syrup or rose-hip syrup when making a crumble or mousse.
3   Add tinned tomatoes to a fresh vegetable casserole or to a vegetable sauce to serve with pasta or rice.
4   Mix tinned peaches or pineapple with orange juice or slices of fresh citrus fruit.
5   Include a tomato salad or a fresh fruit salad in meals where the main dish is something like macaroni cheese, hot dog or beefburger in a bun.

Things to do

1   *Try to find out which foods are fortified with vitamins A and D. Which groups of people are these intended for. Why is it a good idea for these foods to be fortified?*

2   *How do most people get their supply of vitamin D?*

3   *Explain the relationship between carotene and vitamin A. How can you tell which foods contain the most carotene?*

4   *Think up some more ways of improving the vitamin C content of meals. Try out your ideas in your practical classes.*

5   *Look at the fruit juices sold in shops which claim they contain certain amounts of vitamin C. Make a list of the amount each make says it contains and how much it costs. Try to decide which is the best buy. How does the price of each product compare with the price of any fresh fruit which supplies a similar amount of vitamin C?*

1.8 Minerals

Minerals are the other group of nutrients which protect the body and regulate its functions. There are many minerals present in our bodies. The main ones which have to be supplied in food are calcium, phosphorus, iron, sulphur, potassium, sodium, chlorine, magnesium and fluorine.

What do minerals do?

Minerals do three jobs:

1   They help to make *bones* and *teeth*. The main minerals for this are calcium, phosphorus and magnesium.
2   They help to control the *amount of water* in the body. The main minerals for this are sodium, chlorine, potassium, magnesium and phosphorus.
3   They help to make **red blood cells** which are essential for carrying oxygen round the body. The main mineral for this is iron.

Some facts about minerals

The table opposite shows the different minerals and the foods in which they are found. Phosphorus is not included in the table because it is present in most foods. A person who eats a variety of food is never in any danger of not getting enough. The function of phosphorus is the same as calcium. The two minerals work together in the body.

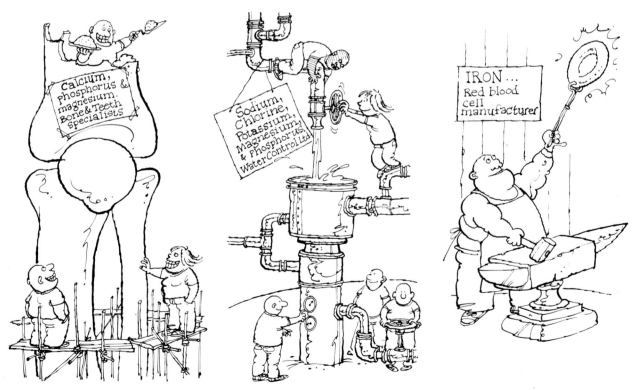

Mineral	Food sources	Functions
Calcium	Milk, cheese, fortified flour, green vegetables, bones in canned sardines and salmon	Forms the structure of bones and teeth. Helps to control the formation of muscles.
Sodium	Common salt, seafood, vegetables	These two together control the amount of water in the body.
Potassium	Meat, fish, fruit, vegetables	
Iron	Meat, bread, flour, other cereal products, potatoes, vegetables	Helps to form **haemoglobin** in red blood cells which carries oxygen needed for energy production.
Iodine	Tap water, seafood, vegetables, iodized salt	Small amounts needed to produce **thyroxine** which helps the thyroid gland work properly.
Fluorine	Fluoridated tap water, seafood, tea	Helps to form strong enamel on teeth.

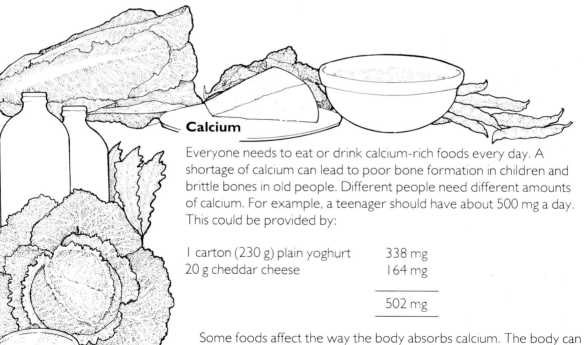

Calcium

Everyone needs to eat or drink calcium-rich foods every day. A shortage of calcium can lead to poor bone formation in children and brittle bones in old people. Different people need different amounts of calcium. For example, a teenager should have about 500 mg a day. This could be provided by:

1 carton (230 g) plain yoghurt	338 mg
20 g cheddar cheese	164 mg
	502 mg

Some foods affect the way the body absorbs calcium. The body can only absorb calcium if it has enough vitamin D. There is an acid in bran, nuts and pulses and another acid in spinach and some other vegetables which can mix with the calcium and produce a salt which is insoluble. This means that the calcium cannot be absorbed into the blood stream and is of no use to our bodies.

19

Iron

It is easier for the body to absorb iron if a food rich in vitamin C is eaten in the same meal. A good example of this would be fried liver with orange slices.

Iron is stored in the liver. Iron from worn out cells can be re-used by the body. This means that it is not absolutely essential for adults to have a daily supply of iron. However, the store of iron in the body must be regularly topped up, so a daily allowance of between 10 and 12 mg is recommended.

If the body does not have enough iron it produces energy more slowly. This leads to tiredness and eventually nutritional anaemia. When bleeding occurs, as in menstruation (periods), it is particularly important to include enough iron-rich food in the diet.

Babies have enough iron in their bodies when they are born to last them about six months. After that age they should be given iron-rich foods to build up their 'store'. Between the ages of 11 and 18 years a recommended daily allowance of iron is 8-12 mg. This could be provided by:

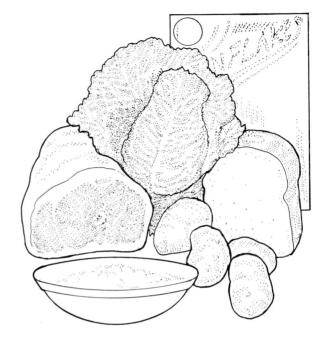

2 lamb's kidneys	10.2 mg
90 g potatoes	0.6 mg
60 g spinach	1.9 mg
	12.7 mg

Gravy made with an oxo cube would increase the amount. So would a cup of cocoa.

Iodine

Some cooking salt, but not all, is fortified with iodine. Fortified salt has **iodized salt** printed on the label. One level teaspoon of iodized salt used in cooking every day will provide enough iodine for one person.

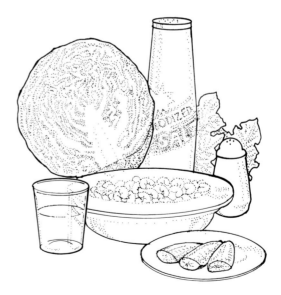

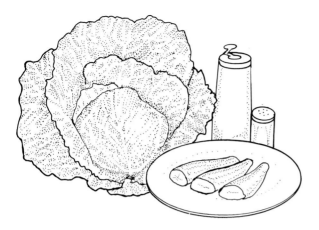

Sodium

Salt contains sodium. People lose it when they sweat. People who work very hard or who live in very hot climates should have extra salt or they may get muscle cramps. However, there is enough salt in the food we eat for most people's needs. People often take more salt than they need by putting extra on their plate.

Fluorine

It is thought that fluorine helps to make tooth enamel stronger and so prevents tooth decay.

Fluoridated drinking water is available in some areas, but not all. Where it is supplied, this is enough for most people's needs.

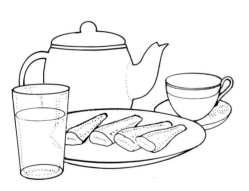

Iron-rich foods

Each of these foods, in these amounts, supplies 4 mg of iron:

1 medium tin sardines or pilchards
8-9 dried figs or apricots
1 large tablespoon treacle
1 rounded teaspoon cocoa
1 rounded teaspoon curry powder
3 rounded tablespoons wholemeal flour
6-7 slices wholemeal bread
2 hamburgers
200 g steak
135 g corned beef
29 g pig's liver
40 g black pudding

Things to do

1 *How could a shortage of calcium affect*
   a *old people,*
   b *children?*

2 *Plan meals for a whole day. Underline the calcium-rich foods.*

3 *Look up recipes which use some of the iron-rich foods mentioned in the box. Prepare a chart showing the recipes which you consider to be:*
   a *popular,*
   b *cheap,*
   c *made with easily available ingredients. Display the chart in the home economics room. Make it eye-catching by including a picture of the finished dish if you can.*

4 *Name four foods which are fortified with either vitamins or minerals or both. Say which minerals and vitamins are included and suggest reasons for this.*

21

Recap I

Complete the following sentences:

1 The names of the nutrient groups are

_____.

2 The two types of protein are _____.

3 Fats are used for _____.

4 Vitamins _____ and _____ are fat
   soluble.

5 Vitamins _____ and _____ are water
   soluble.

Answer these questions with one or more
sentences:

6 What is 'fortification'?

7 What do minerals do?

8 What is textured vegetable protein? Why is it
   useful?

9 What are the advantages of combining two or
   more sources of lower biological protein
   together in the same meal? Give two
   examples of dishes where this is done.

10 Why is it bad planning to have a lot of protein
   food one day and none the next? Give two
   reasons.

11 What sources of energy can the body use?

12 What two things does food do?

13 Keep a record for a week of all the food you
   eat and all the activities that you carry out. See
   if the food you eat balances with the energy
   you use. Try and keep a record for other
   members of your family too. Does everyone
   use the same amount of energy? Eat the same
   amount and type of food? Does the age or
   sex of the person make any difference?

14 Suggest a variety of vitamin-C-rich foods
   which could be included in menus for
   a breakfast,
   b a midday meal,
   c an evening meal.

15 It is sometimes difficult for our bodies to
   absorb iron. Remember that eating a vitamin-
   C-rich food at the same time helps the body
   to use the iron. Try out the following recipes
   in your practical classes. They are all examples
   of meals combining vitamin C and iron.
   a Gingerbread made with treacle and
      served with fresh orange or grapefruit
      juice.
   b Curries served with 'sambals' (side dishes)
      of fresh, raw fruit and vegetables. For
      example, tomato and onion salad with
      lemon juice dressing; peppers
      marinated (soaked) in oil and vinegar
      dressing;
      thinly sliced orange and chive salad.
   c Liver sauté with pilaff and orange salad.

16 Use the *Manual of Nutrition* to calculate the
   energy per portion for the following dishes:
   a *Victoria sandwich cake*
      100 g SR flour
      100 g caster sugar
      100 g soft margarine
      1-2 tablespoons warm water
      2 tablespoons raspberry jam for filling
      1 tablespoon icing sugar to sprinkle on top
   b *Cheese scones*
      200 g plain flour
      4 level teaspoons baking powder
      ½ teaspoon salt
      40 g margarine
      140 ml milk
      50 g grated Edam cheese
      Pinch cayenne pepper

2 Planning and balancing meals

2.1 A balanced diet

When you are planning meals you should try to include enjoyable and varied dishes. Attractive nutritious meals do not just happen they have to be planned.

Planning meals

There are several things you should think about when you are planning meals:

1. The *balance* of a meal — each ingredient from the recipe for good health (page 5) should be found in at least one food in a balanced meal.
2. The *ages* and *occupations* of the people who are going to eat the meal — not everyone needs the same amount of nutrients.
3. The *climate* and *time of year* — in cold weather people prefer warming food. They might not be pleased with cold meat and salad.
4. The food *likes* and *dislikes* of the people — a good cook should try to provide food people like and also encourage them to be adventurous in their eating.
5. The *cost* of food — it is cheaper to buy food that is in season.
6. The *presentation* of food — it should be attractive and colourful, not monotonous. Varied well-garnished and tasty dishes will not bore people, sausage and chips every Tuesday may.
7. The *texture* of food — this should be varied. A meal should not consist of all smooth or all crunchy food, but a mixture of the two.
8. The *time* and *energy* you have for preparing the food.
9. The *flavours* and *temperature* of food — this should also be varied. Do not serve the same flavour or type of dish more than once in a meal.
10. The *colour* of food — try to use brightly-coloured food and see that the different colours blend.

Things to do

1. *Complete the following to make a balanced meal:*
   a *Roast beef, Yorkshire pudding, roast potatoes, peas, _____.*
   b *_____, chappati, dhal, _____.*
   c *Liver casserole, baked potatoes in jackets, casseroled carrots, _____.*
   d *Cornish pasties, _____.*
   e *_____, Brussels sprouts, creamed potatoes, stewed apple, _____.*
   Give your reasons for choosing the dishes you suggested to complete each meal.

2. *How does the meal in the photo score against the 10 points listed above?*

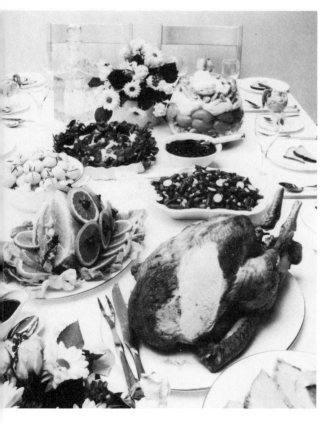

2.2 Special needs

When you plan meals you need to bear in mind the special needs of the people you are cooking for. The following are examples of people with special needs:

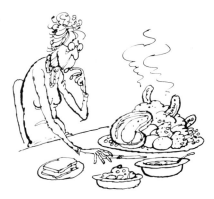

1 **Active people**, such as building workers, miners and athletes, need a lot of energy-giving foods and foods rich in the B group vitamins. Less active people, such as bank clerks, need less.
2 **Young children** need more body-building foods and protective foods than adults.
3 **Elderly people** usually move about less and so they need less energy-giving foods, though they must still have enough body-building and protective foods. Vitamin C is especially important to prevent scurvy which some elderly people suffer from even today. There is more about the needs of the elderly on page 38.

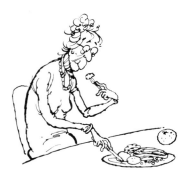

4 **Expectant and nursing mothers** need extra calcium and iron to make the baby's bones, teeth and red blood cells develop properly. These are sometimes taken in supplements such as pills because the mother may not eat enough iron or calcium-rich food in her normal diet to provide the baby with the amount it needs.
5 **Women and girls** who are menstruating must have enough iron-rich food to replace the red blood cells they lose.

Things to do

1 *Write down what is wrong with the following meals and say how they could be improved:*

a *White vegetable soup* *Steamed fish, white sauce* *Creamed potatoes* *Rice pudding*	b **Meal for a teenager** *Fried fish* *Fried potatoes* *Jam tart*	c **Meal for a** **road-construction worker** *Grapefruit* *Lamb chop* *Peas, potatoes* *Fruit salad*
d **Meal for a hot summer's day** *Steak and kidney pudding* *Potatoes, carrots* *Steamed jam sponge, custard*	e **Midday meal for an office worker** *Brown stew and dumplings* *Parsnips, potatoes* *Apple pie, custard*	f *Sausages* *Chips* *Steamed pudding, jam sauce*

2 *Think up some more examples of people with special needs. What would be a good meal to give them?*

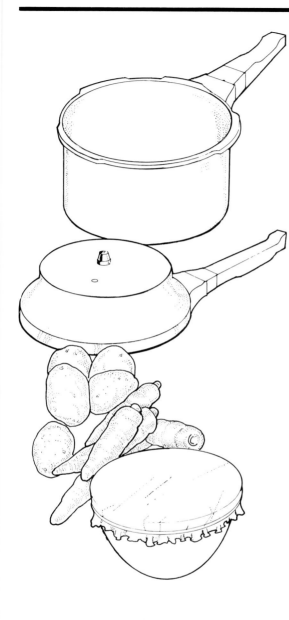

2.3 Saving fuel

Another thing we must think about when planning menus is how we can be economical in our use of fuel. Here are some suggestions as to how you might do this:

1   Try to plan meals so that, if the oven is used, *all* the dishes are cooked in it. This will save fuel.
2   Try making a complete meal using one burner only. You can do this by using a pressure cooker or steamer.

Things to do

1   *Look at the meals below and say with reasons which will save fuel; then give a fuel saving meal of your own.*

a *Toad-in-the-hole*
   Jacket potatoes
   Stuffed onions
   Rhubarb crumble
   Custard

b *Chicken pie*
   Creamed potatoes
   Peas
   Lemon pancakes

c *Scotch eggs*
   Salad
   Potatoes in jackets
   Apple pie

d *Steamed fish*
   Parsley sauce
   potatoes and carrots
   Steamed jam sponge pudding
   Custard

2   *Think of a well-balanced main meal which uses either a pressure cooker or a steamer.*

3   *Think of some more examples of meals that save fuel. Try cooking them in a lesson or at home.*

2.4 Meal patterns

Meal patterns vary from one family to another and often from one part of the country to another. From a nutritional point of view it does not matter when food is eaten. The important thing is for people to get the right amounts of the right kinds of food. This will ensure that their nutritional needs are fulfilled and their hunger is satisfied. They will also enjoy their food better.

It is usually convenient for people to have a routine for their eating. Each group of people develops its own eating pattern to suit its own particular needs.

There is no 'correct' pattern for meals. Normally in Britain we have breakfast, a midday meal and an evening meal. The evening meal could be a high tea or dinner, depending on whether it is the main meal of the day or not.

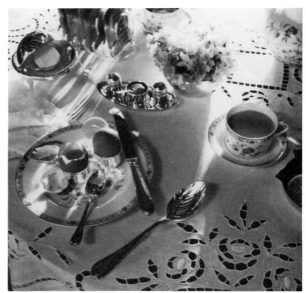

Boiled egg for a breakfast

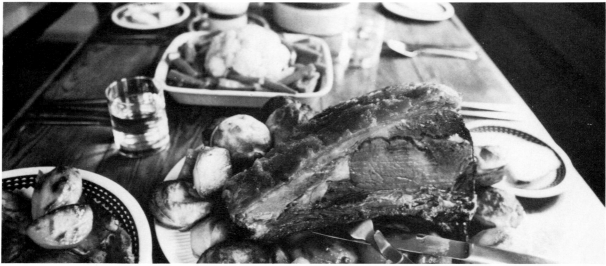

Roast meat for a special meal when everyone is at home.

Things to do

1 *When do you have your main meal of the day? Why is it at this time? Discuss in your group to see if anyone has a different pattern from yours. Is the main meal of the day the only time when everyone is at home together and when there is a chance to talk?*

2 *Find out about meal patterns in other countries. In what ways are they the same or different to our meal patterns?*

2.5 Breakfast

This is an important meal which is sometimes neglected. Adults work more efficiently and safely and school pupils are more attentive and receptive if they eat breakfast at the start of their day.

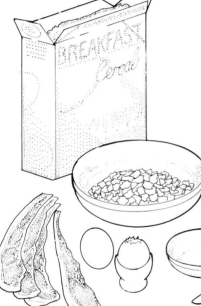

During sleep the body is resting and just 'ticking over'. In the morning food provides energy to start the day's activities. Food also prevents 'hunger pangs' which can lead to nibbling between meals.

You might have hunger pangs around mid-morning if you have missed breakfast. Mid-morning it is usually more convenient to eat something quick such as a biscuit or a bar of chocolate. This is poor nutrition and is also bad for your teeth.

Some facts about breakfast

1 A good breakfast should supply about a quarter of the daily food needs of most people.
2 Some breakfast cereals have extra nutrients added when they are being made. This makes them especially valuable nutritionally. Some nutrients are lost when breakfast cereals are manufactured and these are replaced in fortified cereals.
3 Fruit juices and cereals with milk make good breakfast food. The cereals provide the quick burst of energy you need to start the day.
4 Time is short, so the food must be quick and easy to prepare. Poached, boiled or fried eggs with bacon are all suitable breakfast dishes.
5 There are some people who cannot face eating breakfast, sometimes because they have to get up too early. It is important then to see that they get all the nutrients they need in their other meals.

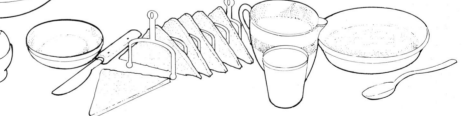

Things to do

1 *Look at packets of cereals and note what nutrients they contain. Look at a number of different kinds. Do they all contain the same nutrients?*

2 *Look back at your investigation of fortified fruit drinks (page 17). Would any of these be valuable at breakfast time? If so, why?*

3 *Prepare a time plan for the preparation of a good breakfast. Show how to 'dove-tail' (fit in) the other things you have to do in getting ready for work or school.*

Breakfast time Plan

7·30 a.m. get up

7·40 a.m. wash

7·55 a.m. breakfast

Menu

Breakfast
Orange juice
Muesli
Wholemeal toast and
    marmalade
Tea

Midday Meal
?

Evening meal
Grapefruit
Rolled fillets of plaice
    in mushroom sauce
Boiled potatoes and peas
Apple pie and custard

2.6 Midday meal

The midday meal is usually a 'quick meal' during the working week. It can be a packed meal taken to work or school. Here are some important points to remember:

1 The food should carry you through to evening meal time. You shouldn't want snacks or other food in between time.
2 Active people, growing children and teenagers need more at midday than other people.
3 The meal should include between a quarter and a third of the day's food from the ingredients in the recipe for good health (page 5).
4 When planning a midday meal bear in mind what was eaten at breakfast and what will be eaten later in the day.

Packed lunches

Some important points:

1 If you are making up a packed lunch every day, try to make each one slightly different.
2 Use food which *packs* and *travels well*, so that it is appetizing and attractive to eat.
3 Try not to include more sugary and starchy foods than the person needs.
4 Do not make the packed lunch too *heavy* or *inconvenient* to carry.
5 Make the food *easy to eat* without a knife and fork.
6 Provide food with different *textures*. Make sure some crisp food such as an apple, is included.
7 Packed lunches can be rather dry, so try to include a drink or a juicy fruit.
8 Sandwiches can be prepared for a whole week and deep frozen. They should be wrapped in foil to stop them drying. Label each pack with the date it was made and the filling you put in.

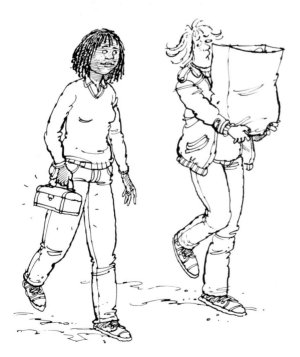

Here are some examples of different packed lunches you could prepare:

1. Home-made soup in a flask with cheese straws and an apple.
2. Wholemeal bread sandwiches with some protein food filling, e.g. cheese and pickle, peanut butter, sardine and apple.
3. Savoury quiche with carrot and celery.
4. Cold meat and a tomato with fruit and nut bread.

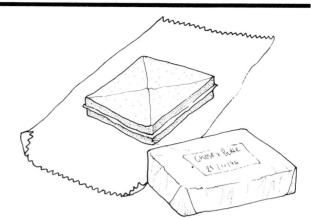
Preparing sandwiches for the freezer

Canteen meals

People have very different tastes when choosing food. Many canteens try to suit most tastes by serving a variety of foods. This often makes it difficult to choose. Take care to choose the right food for your needs. Choose food that will enable you to do a good afternoon's work.

For example, if you usually use a lot of energy in the morning, your midday meal should include plenty of energy-giving food so that you can work well without getting tired. If, on the other hand, your work is more sedentary (you are mainly sitting down) a heavy meal with a lot of sugary and starchy food may make you sleepy in the afternoon. It would therefore be better to choose less bulky, more concentrated food such as toasted sandwiches or minestrone soup and a roll, followed by some fresh fruit.

Midday meal at home

This should be a light meal if you have your main meal of the day in the evening. The following meals could be eaten at midday, or, if this is the main meal of the day, they could be served as tea or supper:

1. Hot foods e.g. spaghetti bolognaise, hamburgers, macaroni cheese, fish pie with a tossed salad.
2. Soup and toasted sandwiches.
3. Open sandwiches e.g. cold meat, fish, cheese with salad.

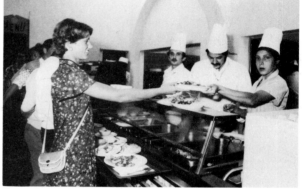
Queueing up in a canteen

Things to do

1. *Make a list of sandwiches and fillings suitable for preparation in bulk and deep freezing.*

2. *Look at the types of convenience foods available. Report on their flavours and prices and the advantages of using them. What nutritional advantage would there be in using milk to reconstitute dried soup rather than water? (Look at page 60 to check facts about milk.)*

3. *Find out about the different ways of packing lunches and the materials that are used. Try some simple tests to see how well they work. Are the materials greaseproof, waterproof, easily crushed? Compare the costs of the various materials.*

2.7 **The main meal of the day**

This can be at midday or in the evening. In most families it is the only time the people can all meet and talk together, so the meal is a sociable occasion.

The meal can have two or three courses. It will often include soup or another appetizer, a main course and a dessert or fruit and cheese.

The main dish should include some protein food. (Look back to pages 7 to 9 to remind yourself about protein.) It is best to combine food sources of higher and lower biological value protein. Good examples of this are chilli con carne, moussaka, meat pie and lasagne. They make a very nutritious main course. They can be served with a salad or vegetables.

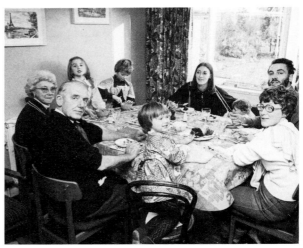
The main meal of the day is often a sociable occasion

Planning

If you plan all your main meals for a week ahead it can help you to balance the food budget. Planning will also help you to practise good nutrition and you will be able to make the meals you serve more varied and interesting.

Forward planning helps the cook to know what shopping and advance meal preparation is needed. These can be fitted into the day's activities so that they do not all have to be done when the working day is over and everyone is tired and hungry.

Saving time and energy

Here are some tips for saving time and energy:

1 Use a pressure cooker, microwave oven, slow cooker or an oven with an automatic time switch.
2 Prepare food in bulk and freeze it. For example, make double the quantity you need of a basic minced meat recipe and freeze half for another time.
3 Make sensible use of convenience foods.
4 Occasionally buy take-away foods such as fish and chips, Chinese meals or beefburgers and 'French fries'.

There is nothing wrong with using convenience foods and take-away foods from time to time, if it is not done too often and if some fresh fruits or vegetables are included in the same meal. For example, a take-away hamburger with French fries followed by an orange or an apple would be a reasonable meal.

Things to do

1 *List the advance preparations a busy cook could make so that the main meal of the day could be cooked and served quickly.*

2 *Notice the variety of convenience foods for main meal dishes next time you are out shopping. Read the contents label of each one. Think of the fresh foods you could include in a meal in which you are using one of these foods.*

2.8 Shops and shopping

We have thought about the foods we like to eat and the meals we enjoy and we have learnt how to get a balanced diet from these foods. Now it is time we went shopping.

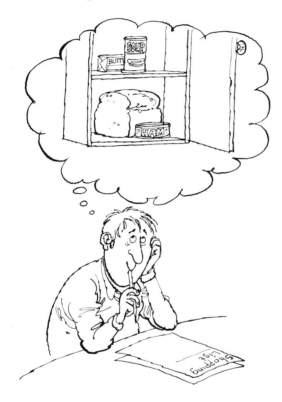

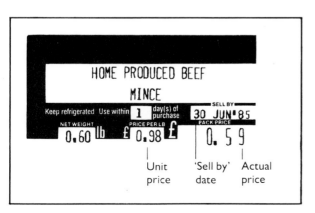

Before you go

Food is expensive so it is important to get good value for money. Here is a list of things to do before going shopping which will help you make sure your budget balances:

1 Work out how much money you have for food — remember to put some aside to pay the milk bill.
2 *Plan the menus* for the week — remember to include some economy meals.
3 Check the store cupboard and make a list of food you need to buy.
4 *Calculate* roughly how much your list is going to cost — make some alterations if you haven't enough money.

In the shops

Now to the shops. Here are some helpful tips:

1 *Compare* prices and quality — newspapers, radio and TV have regular items about 'seasonal' and 'good buy' foods.
2 *Never* shop when you are *hungry* — you will always be tempted to buy more than you need!
3 Try to choose a quiet time to shop — you will be able to concentrate more on your list and get through more quickly.
4 Keep your list handy and buy only what is on it — if you have a pocket calculator use it to tot up as you go along.
5 Check the **'sell by' dates** — these are stamped on some perishable foods such as cream. Up to the 'sell by' date the food should be in the best condition.
6 Notice the **unit price** of the food you are buying — this is the price per pound or ½ kilo and it is printed beside the actual price you are paying for the item. It helps you to check you are getting good value for money.
7 Choose shops which have high standards of cleanliness — a shop with a dirty floor and untidy assistants is not a good place to buy food.

31

Where to shop

After a few visits to a high street you will get to know the best shops for you. There are several types to choose from:

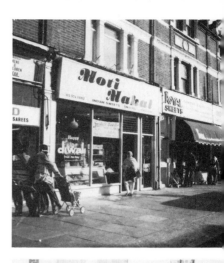

1 **Supermarkets** — these carry a wide range of goods. They are often owned by a large company.
2 **General stores** — these are smaller versions of supermarkets and are often found in country areas. They may be owned by the shopkeeper or rented to him or her by a big co-operative such as Spar or Mace. Sometimes these shops act as the Post Office as well.
3 **Corner shops** — these carry a fairly wide range of foods and may be the nearest shop to your house. They are often owned by the shopkeeper and are often open for much longer each day than other shops.
4 **Specialist shops** — these sell one type of merchandise only, such as fish, meat or vegetables.
5 **Chain and department stores** — these carry a wide range of goods including food.
6 **Hypermarkets** — these are very big supermarkets where you can buy most things from pins to caravans and cars. They are often outside towns and always have a large car park.
7 **Street markets** — these are rows of stalls in some streets. Food prices at the stalls are sometimes lower than in shops, but *not always*. Be sure to check price and quality carefully.

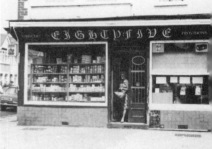

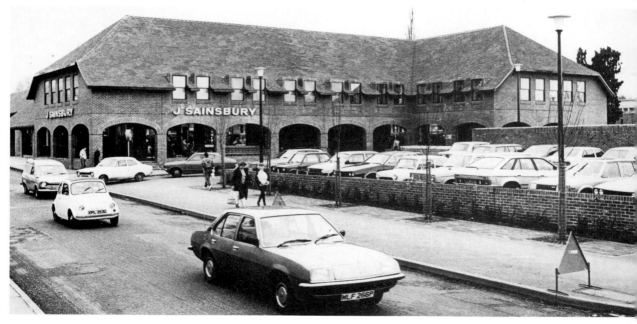

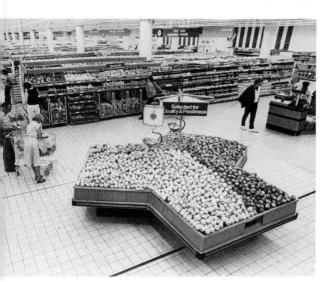

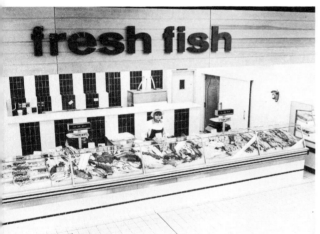

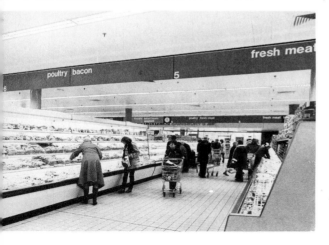

Choosing the kind of shop

The choice is really between the large supermarkets with a wide range of goods where you can do all the shopping under one roof, and the smaller specialist shops where you get more personal attention. Each has advantages and disadvantages.

Supermarkets

Advantages

1 A wide choice of food is available, including 'own brands' which are often cheaper.
2 Food is presented in a bright, hygienic and orderly way.
3 There may be bargain offers.
4 There is often a large car park just outside with wheeled trolleys to carry food to the car.

Disadvantages

1 There is a temptation to spend too much money.
2 Fresh food such as meat and vegetables is often already weighed and wrapped, so you may not be able to find the amount and exact kind you want.
3 There may be queues at the checkout.
4 It is difficult to check prices as the cashier rings them up on the till. Mistakes *are* sometimes made.
5 Walking around a big store can be tiring.

Smaller shops

Advantages

1 Personal attention — the shopkeeper may know what the family likes and will recommend good buys to suit their tastes.
2 Food can sometimes be delivered.
3 The service is friendly.

Disadvantages

1 There is less choice of goods and often no bargain offers.
2 Prices may be slightly higher.
3 Goods may be past their best because they may not be sold very quickly.

Other ways of shopping for food

There are other ways of shopping for food. One of these is **bulk buying**. This is buying large quantities at a reduced price. If you have enough money for the initial outlay and enough storage space this is usually a very economical way of buying food. For example, meat bought in large quantities is very much cheaper, but of course you need to have a freezer to store it in.

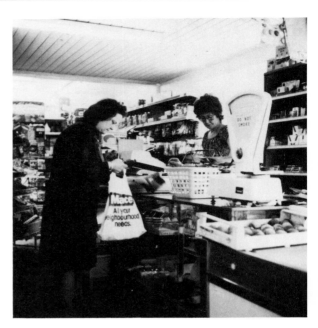

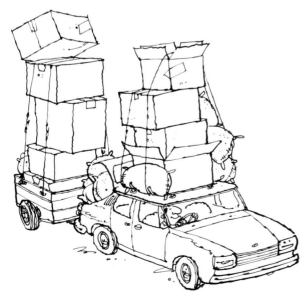

Things to do

1 *Plan menus for your family for a week. Make a shopping list of the food you will need. Find out the prices for the things on the list at your local shops. Compare the prices at two different shops if you can.*

2 *If the shopkeepers have time to spare, ask them about people's shopping habits. Which foods do they sell most of? Are people influenced by television advertising? Think up some more questions.*

3 *Think about the advantages and disadvantages of bulk buying. Discuss them with your group. Find out if there is a 'cash and carry' warehouse near the school. Try to arrange a visit to see what sort of goods they sell and in what quantities. Take a pocket calculator with you and use it to find out if the bulk price is cheaper than the price in the shops (the* **retail** *price).*

Recap 2

Are the following sentences true or false?

1 The ages and occupations of people who are going to eat a meal are not important.
2 It is a good idea to serve several dishes of the same colour in the same meal e.g. carrot soup as the first course and stewed apricots and custard for pudding.
3 Elderly people do not need a lot of energy-giving food.
4 Active people need a lot of vitamin A.
5 Expectant and nursing mothers need extra calcium and iron.

Answer these questions:

6 How much of our daily food needs should breakfast supply?
7 What are the four important points to remember about a midday meal?
8 Which nutrient should the main dish of the main meal of the day include?
9 How can a cook save time and energy? Give as many different ways as you can.
10 What is a 'sell by' date?
11 What is a 'unit price'?

12 Plan a meal for your family. Think about the points mentioned on page 23. Explain your choice of meal. Use the following words in your answer:
Ages and occupations...time of year...cost...presentation.

13 When you next visit the greengrocer or go to the supermarket, find out what the following vegetables are, how much they cost and at what time of the year they are cheapest:
Courgettes...Chinese leaves...chicory...aubergines...broccoli...spinach...
Jerusalem
artichokes...peppers...leeks...marrows.
How can each be prepared, cooked and used in meals?

14 In your group, organize a study of food shopping habits. You could do this by making up a questionnaire for people to fill in or you could have a list of questions to ask people in the street. Ask questions like these:
Where do you buy your food?
What type of shop do you prefer to buy food from?
What type of shop do you never buy food from?
How often do you go shopping for food?
Think up some more questions of your own.
    Get information from as many people as you can. Which type of shop is most popular in your area? Do most people use just one type of shop or do they use several different shops? Does age make a difference to shopping habits?

15 A girl of 16 chose the following meal from the school canteen at midday:
50 g baked beans on
38 g toasted bread
12 g butter
100 g apple
70 ml milk in a cup of coffee
Plan a suitable breakfast and evening meal for this girl to eat on the same day as this midday canteen meal.

3 Diets and health

3.1 Vegetarians

Vegetarians never eat meat or fish, often for moral or religious reasons. There are two types of vegetarian — vegans and lacto-vegetarians.

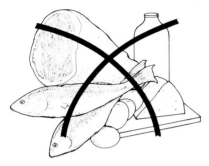

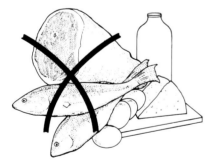

Vegans

Vegans are very strict vegetarians who avoid all animals products. They will not eat meat, fish, cheese, eggs or milk, so it can be difficult for them to make sure they are getting all the correct nutrients. They should have enough protein if they eat soya beans and a mixture of proteins of lower biological value from nuts, peas and other types of beans. However, they may be short of the essential amino acids if they do not plan their meals carefully. (See page 7 to remind you about this.)

Vegans' diets are **bulky** because they have to eat a lot of food to get enough nutrients. Many of the nutrients come from vegetables. These are low in energy value, so very active vegans must make up for this by eating plenty of bread, pasta and potatoes.

It may be difficult for vegans to get enough calcium, iron, B group vitamins and vitamin D from plant products alone. However, a diet-conscious vegan can get round this problem with a little thought. Yeast extract is a very good non-animal source of B group vitamins. Vegans can use it to make gravy and stock. The various texturized vegetable protein products are useful too, especially if the manufacturers fortify them with iron and B group vitamins. Vegans' diets are now more interesting, as today there are a lot of recipe books available for them.

Lacto-vegetarians

Lacto-vegetarians will eat eggs, cheese and milk, so it is much easier to provide a nutritionally well-balanced diet for them. Remember that yeast extract must be used to make gravy and stock rather than meat stock cubes.

Things to do

1 *Think up a meal for a lacto-vegetarian. How could you adapt it for a vegan? Use recipe books to help you.*

2 *Look in your local shops to see what kinds of nuts, peas and beans are available. Try out some recipes which use them in your practical classes.*

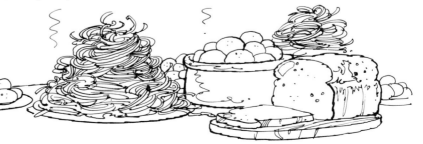

3.2 Some ethnic groups

Some ethnic groups in the UK may have special nutritional difficulties. When people come to the UK they may want to follow their traditional diets and customs but the different conditions in the UK mean that they may no longer get all the nutrients they need.

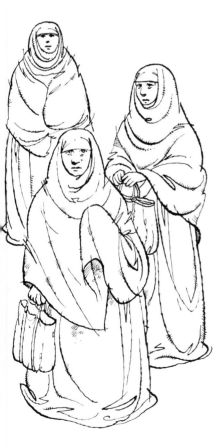

Some Asians in the UK do not have enough vitamin D in their traditional diets to prevent rickets (in children) and osteomalacia (in adults). Of course we don't just get our vitamin D from food sources. We also get it from sunlight acting on the skin. However, some Asian women, for example Sikhs and Muslims, cover their whole body with clothes. In our climate this means that they do not have enough sunlight on their skin and so they do not make enough vitamin D. Some Muslim and Hindu women stay indoors a lot and this also cuts down the amount of vitamin D their bodies make.

There have also been cases of **nutritional anaemia** in Asians, caused by a shortage of iron. This is because some Asians do not eat meat or eggs.

Some foods can interfere with iron absorbtion. These are called **inhibitors**. Wholemeal flour contains an inhibitor called **phytic acid**.

What can be done?

People used to a different diet and way of life, who come to live in the UK, can make sure they get the necessary amount of nutrients by remembering the following:

1 Vegetable oil margarine can be used instead of the fat called ghee often used by Asians for cooking. Margarine is fortified with vitamins A and D.
2 Vitamin D supplements are available for all children up to five years old and for pregnant and lactating women.
3 Fortified soya bean products can be used in food to prevent nutritional anaemia.
4 If iron is lacking, people could use yeast with wholemeal flour recipes, as the yeast lessens the effect of the inhibitor.

Things to do

1 *Find out about the traditional diets of some ethnic groups known to you. In what ways are they similar or different to your own diet? Do you think all the diets have enough vitamin D in them?*

2 *Design a poster to warn people of the danger of not having enough vitamin D. Make your poster as visual as possible. You could include pictures of the diseases caused by a lack of vitamin D. You could also say how to make sure you do get enough of the vitamins.*

3.3 Elderly people

Most people are less active as they grow older. This means they use less energy, so they should eat less of the foods which supply mostly energy (e.g. sugar which provides only energy). However, they must take care that they do not lose weight.

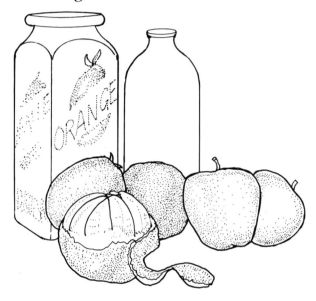

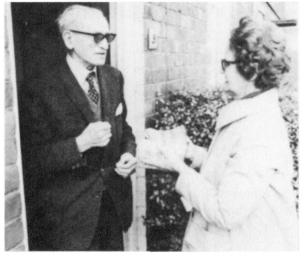

A meals on wheels delivery

Elderly people need a daily supply of vitamin C just like everyone else. This can easily be provided by an orange, an apple or a fortified fruit drink.

People's bones get more brittle as they grow older, so they need plenty of vitamin-D-rich foods such as herring, mackerel, cod-liver oil and malt and calcium from foods such as milk.

What special problems can old people have?

Some old people have other problems which may stop them eating properly. Some examples are:

1 Loneliness and depression — meals on wheels and luncheon clubs may help this.
2 Immobility or handicap — a good neighbour may be able to help by shopping for the old person. Ready-prepared foods can also help, especially if the person has arthritis or has restricted movement.
3 Loose and ill-fitting dentures — this can make it difficult to chew properly. The dentist can put this right.
4 Money — old people may not be able to afford the foods they need.

In spite of these difficulties, there is no special diet for old age. Many elderly people stay healthy and active all their lives and have a healthy interest in food.

All food for elderly people should be easy and quick to prepare. Foods which are rich sources of nutrients should be used because people tend to eat smaller quantities of food as they grow older.

Things to do

1 *Plan meals for an elderly person for a week. Think about the following: Cost…appearance…bulk…vitamins… preparation.*

2 *Think of some more problems which may stop old people from eating properly. How could they be solved?*

3.4 People living alone

Many young people leave home to work, or to study and have to look after themselves for the first time. Sometimes they are careless about their diet because they are too busy or cannot be bothered. Not eating properly can make people feel tired and ill, so it is worth taking a little trouble to make sure they are eating enough of the right kind of food.

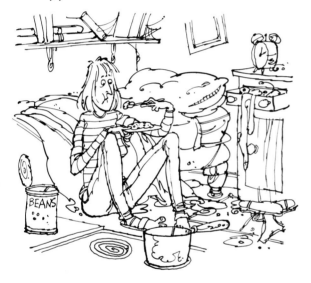

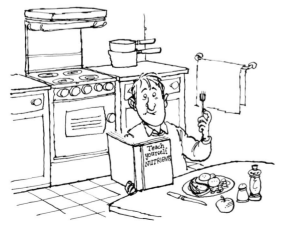

You can use the wide range of convenience foods and take-away foods available, provided some fresh food is also included. This is easily done by eating fresh fruit every day and sometimes having a salad with the main dish.

It is useful to know something about nutrients and what they do for you, as well as about preparing and cooking simple meals. This enables you to have a balanced diet and also gives you the satisfaction of being independent for the first time.

Quick and easy cooking

Here are some ways people living alone can have a good meal without too much trouble:

1 Use the grill for a whole meal. For example, serve grilled chops, tomatoes and mushrooms with watercress and potato crisps, followed by grilled banana sprinkled with brown sugar.
2 Beat up an egg in milk for a hurried breakfast.
3 Make soup from a packet or tin and serve it with cheese on toasted wholemeal bread, followed by an apple.
4 Make use of prepared mixes. For example, use frozen pastry for meat pies or fresh fruit pies.
5 Use 'cook-in' sauces to make nutritious, tasty dishes from fresh ingredients.

Things to do

1 *What other things can you do to have a good meal if you live alone?*

2 *Write a menu for yourself for one day. Include convenience food and fresh food in some of the meals.*

3 *Investigate the foods available in your local supermarket for people living alone. Is it possible to buy individual portions of most foods or is most food sold in packs containing more than one portion?*

3.5 People on a small budget

It is difficult to meet nutritional needs and satisfy hunger when money is short. It is tempting to buy too much sugary food because this is both filling and cheap.

Here are a few ways round this problem:

1   If you have a garden, grow your own vegetables and fruit. A lot can be grown on a small piece of ground. Read the instructions on the seed packets and time your planting of seeds so you have something to harvest all year round.
2   Buy food when it is in season.
3   Learn about cheaper cuts of meat and how to prepare and cook them to make sure they are tender. A pressure cooker would be a good investment for this.
4   Find out about meat extenders and cheap alternatives to meat, such as textured vegetable protein products. Learn how to prepare and present them attractively.

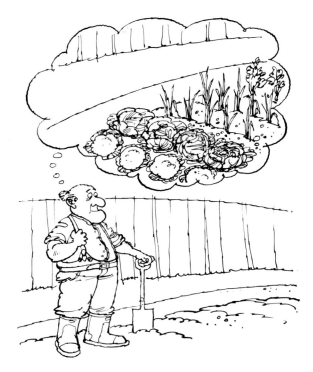

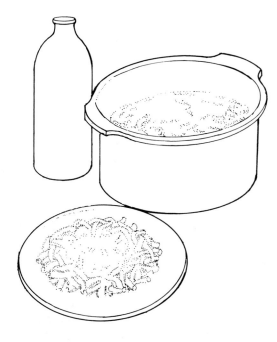

5   Include 'economy' dishes which are nutritious, such as macaroni cheese, or bean and tomato casserole. Meat is expensive and you do not need to eat it at every meal.
6   Do not cut down on the amount of milk you drink. Milk provides valuable nutrients for a low cost (see page 60). Use it in cooking as well as for drinking.

Things to do

1   *Think of some more ways round the problem of having little money.*

2   *Collect as many recipes as you can which use minced meat. Try out some of them in your practical classes.*

3   *Think of some more 'economy' dishes. Work out how much each one would cost to make for a family of four. Remember that the dishes must contain nutrients from the recipe for good health.*

3.6 People recovering from an illness

People recovering from an illness are called convalescents. They need a special diet to help them get well quickly and to help them return to normal, healthy eating. People recovering from severe illnesses need special care as they are often very weak. It is best to start by giving them small amounts of food. Then you can gradually increase the amount of food. Foods such as eggs and milk are good to help repair the body.

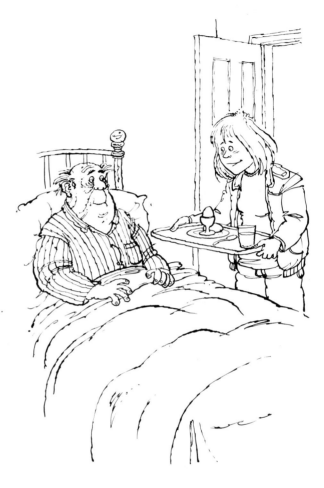

Rules to remember

1 Convalescents should have plenty of liquids to stop **dehydration** — make sure the patient always has a drink available.
2 Food should be simple, well-cooked and attractively served — this will help tempt the patient's appetite.
3 Avoid fried and rich foods — appetite and digestion are not very good after an illness.
4 Give the patient lots of small meals rather than a few large ones — this will encourage the patient to eat more.
5 Include some raw fruit and vegetables every day — this will provide the convalescent with essential vitamins and will also help digestion.

Which foods are good for convalescents?

The table shows which foods can be given to convalescents and which foods should be avoided.

Suitable foods	Foods to avoid
Eggs	All fried and greasy foods
Milk	Pork and fat meat
Fish	Sausage
Chicken	Rich pastry
Tender meat e.g. lamb	Fresh new bread
Fruit and fresh vegetables	Highly seasoned foods
Soups	Sauces and pickles
Bread	High-sugar foods

Things to do

1 *Plan a day's menu for someone recovering from an illness. Use the table to help you choose suitable foods. Remember that it is best to provide small frequent meals. For example, it might be a good idea for a patient to have a milky drink and a scone mid-morning and a cup of tea and some bread and butter mid-afternoon in addition to cooked meals for lunch and dinner.*

2 *Think of some ways of making meals appealing to convalescents. For example, how could you make the meal tray look decorative?*

3.7 **Over-eating**

What makes people overweight?

As countries in the West have become richer, the people have not always become healthier. People in these countries are less active than they used to be because today they use cars and labour-saving equipment much more. As a result, there are many people in the West who are obese (overweight). Too much food and too little exercise are the main causes of **obesity** — look back to Unit 2 to remind yourself about this.

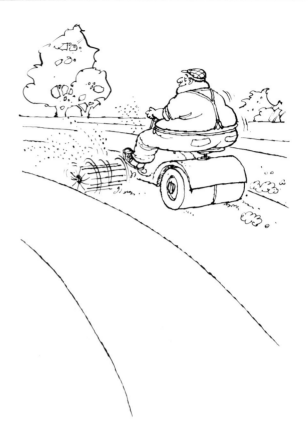

Why obesity is bad

Obesity is not only unattractive and depressing, it is also unhealthy. Overweight people can get breathless because they have a lot of fat to carry around with them. Obesity places extra strain on the heart, and on joints and veins in the legs. **Diabetes** and **gall bladder disease** may be connected with obesity.

Obese people are more likely to have accidents because their weight may make then clumsy.

Losing weight

The energy value of food is measured in kilojoules. Look at the table. It shows food and physical activities which use the same amount of energy. Did you notice that it takes a long time playing golf to 'burn' up 68 g of sugar?

Obesity does not happen overnight. It is caused by eating more food than you burn up. If this happens day after day you will get fat. It also takes time to lose weight.

People who do need to lose weight should eat less for some time, until they reach the right weight for their height and build. To keep to this weight, they need to watch that they don't eat more food than they use up in physical activity.

In adolescence, boys and girls may put on 'puppy' fat. This usually disappears after adolescence so long as the person is eating sensibly. If people

Energy used (1250 kJ)	
Activity	Time
Golf	2 hrs
Tennis	¾-1 hr
Gardening	¾-1 hr
Football	30-40 mins
Competitive swimming Cross-country running Hill climbing	less than 1 hr
4 mile walk	1 hr
Do-it-yourself house repairs and decorating	2 hrs

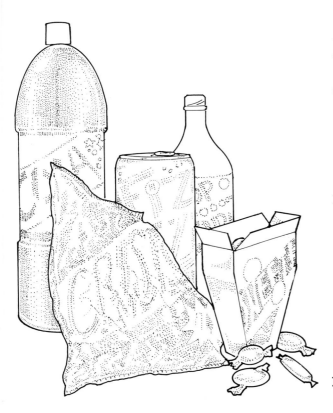

become obsessed with slimming this can lead to the illness **anorexia nervosa**. This is a serious illness in which people feel that their body is fat and that they are overweight no matter how slim they are.

Guidelines for eating

1   Do not consistently over-eat. This confuses the part of your brain that normally tells you when you are hungry. Persistent over-eating can mean that you *feel* hungry even when you do not need more food.

2   Learn to limit the amount of 'empty calories' and 'junk food' you eat. These foods are very easy to buy and are often pleasant to eat. Empty calorie foods have a lot of sugar and supply no other nutrient. Examples are sweets, toffees, candy-floss and fizzy drinks.

Junk food is anything that does not contain many nutrients. Many packaged snacks, such as crisps, are junk food. Eating these too often can spoil your appetite for the meals where you *would* get the essential nutrients.

3   Cut down on fatty foods such as butter, cream and cooking fats. Eat fewer cakes and pastries. These have invisible fats in them.

4   Remember that alcoholic drinks generally supply only energy value. They count as empty calories.

Things to do

1   *Study television and magazine advertisements and note how many are for 'junk foods' or foods containing 'empty calories'. Price these items in the shops. Try to work out the energy value of each one.*

2   *Try out some recipes for slimmers. Think up a menu for a dinner party for people who are trying to lose weight.*

Energy eaten (1250 kJ)	
Food	Quantity
Sugar	70 g or 18 lumps
Bread	6 slices
Milk	450 ml
Cheese	65 g
Bacon	75 g
Eggs	3 large size
Potatoes	500 g
Biscuits	6 digestive biscuits
Gin or whisky	6 single measures
Beer	1 litre
Table wine	½ litre (2 glasses)

3.8 Too much sugar

*Tooth decay (or **dental caries**) is common among young children in the western world. It is caused mainly by eating too many sweet, sticky foods. These stick to the teeth and are then changed into acids by bacteria in the mouth. These acids wear away the enamel of the teeth and cause decay.*

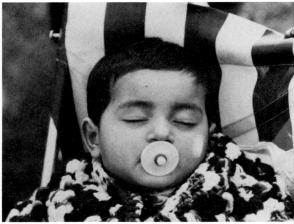

A dummy filled with a sugary drink can harm a baby's teeth

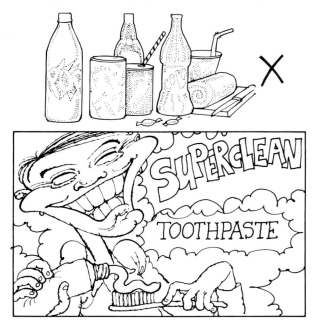

Dental decay can start very early in a child's life if a 'comforter' is given. These comforters, such as a dummy, are sometimes filled with a sugary drink. They are often left in the baby's mouth for a long time. As the baby sucks, the front teeth can be damaged; the child also gets a taste for sweet things.

The message is clear; do not eat too may sweets, and clean your teeth regularly. *Remember:* raw fruit and vegetables can be natural teeth cleaners.

Other points to remember

1 Eating sweet things between meals spoils your appetite for essential foods.
2 Do not eat too may cakes, biscuits, jams and jellies because they do not supply any vitamins from the B group. These vitamins are essential ingredients in the recipe for good health.
3 Sugar supplies 100% energy and no other nutrient.

How to reduce your sugar intake

1 Put less sugar on cereals and fruit.
2 Do not drink too many sweetened drinks, such as cola and fruit squashes. If you are thirsty, drink water or milk or fresh fruit drinks.
3 Eat fresh fruit instead of a pudding.

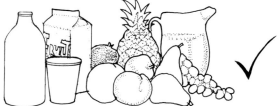

Things to do

1 *Find out as much as you can about tooth decay. What do dentists tell you to do to prevent it?*

2 *How can parents prevent their children from developing a 'sweet tooth'? Give four ways.*

3 *Design an advertisement for a new 'super' toothpaste. Say what your toothpaste will do, that other toothpastes cannot do.*

3.9 Heart disease

The number of people who suffer from this disease has increased since World War II. No one really knows what causes it. Doctors think many things contribute to it. Smoking and not taking enough exercise are two ways people put themselves at risk. Another factor is thought to be eating too much fat, particularly animal fats.

Two kinds of fats

Fats are made up of carbon, hydrogen and oxygen. The carbon part of the fat 'holds' the hydrogen. If the carbon has as much hydrogen as it can hold we say it is **saturated**. If the carbon has room for more hydrogen we say it is **unsaturated**. Saturated fats tend to be those from animal sources. They are found in lard, butter, suet, full fat cheeses such as Cheddar and Brie, and egg yolk. Unsaturated fats usually come from vegetable sources. Examples of foods containing these are sunflower oil, corn oil and safflower oil.

Fats help to produce **cholesterol** in our bodies. Some cholesterol is necessary and is always present in our blood, but there can be too much. When this happens, cholesterol collects in the walls of the blood vessels, especially the coronary arteries, and clogs them up. The coronary arteries take blood to the muscles of the heart itself. If these are clogged up, the heart cannot get enough blood and cannot work properly.

Unsaturated fats make less cholesterol in the body than saturated fats. Some people believe that eating unsaturated fats (instead of saturated fats) *may* help to reduce the risk of coronary heart disease. Can you see why?

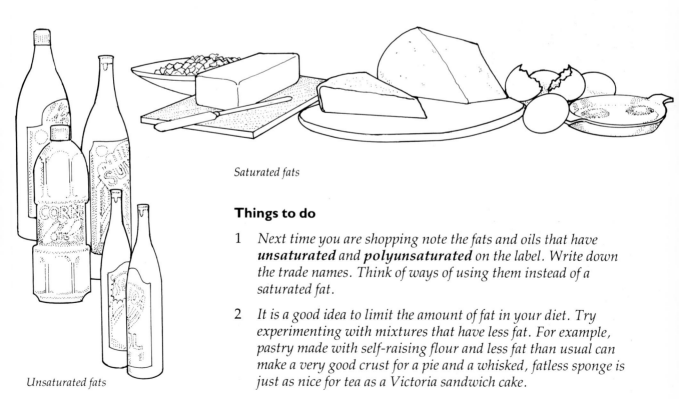

Saturated fats

Unsaturated fats

Things to do

1 *Next time you are shopping note the fats and oils that have **unsaturated** and **polyunsaturated** on the label. Write down the trade names. Think of ways of using them instead of a saturated fat.*

2 *It is a good idea to limit the amount of fat in your diet. Try experimenting with mixtures that have less fat. For example, pastry made with self-raising flour and less fat than usual can make a very good crust for a pie and a whisked, fatless sponge is just as nice for tea as a Victoria sandwich cake.*

3.10 Dietary fibre and bowel disease

Fibre is not digested but it is important because it adds bulk to food. This can prevent constipation and other more serious bowel disorders. Fibre comes from **cellulose** in fruit and vegetables, and from the outer husks of cereals. During digestion the fibre absorbs water and this means that the faeces are soft and bulky and pass easily out of the body in a short space of time.

In refined foods, such as white flour, the outer husk of the grain has been taken away. It is thought that a diet with too much refined food can lead to bowel disorders. The British and Americans eat far less cereal fibre now than they did a hundred years ago. There has been a fashion for eating white bread and polished rice and highly-processed foods. This is now changing and people are using more **whole foods**, that is, rice, flour and cereal with the husk still there.

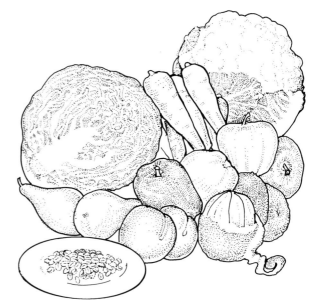

How to eat more fibre

You can get fibre into your diet by

1 eating plenty of fruit and vegetables,
2 eating breakfast cereals that contain bran,
3 using wholemeal flour and eating wholemeal bread,
4 using brown rice, wholemeal pasta and different kinds of nuts.

Things to do

1 *Try out some recipes for cakes using wholemeal flour. (You will find recipes for these in vegetarian cookery books.)*

2 *Organize a 'whole food' exhibition. Display as many whole food ingredients and dishes as you can.*

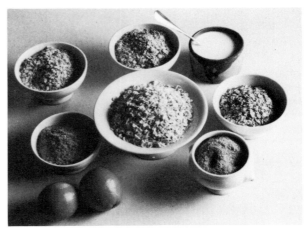

'Whole foods' use unrefined rice, flour and cereals

Recap 3

Pair up the 'heads' and 'tails' of the following sentences correctly:

1 Vegans...have special nutritional difficulties.
2 Lacto-vegetarians...need less sugars and starches.
3 Some ethnic groups...will eat eggs, cheese and milk.
4 Elderly people...should be given frequent small meals.
5 Convalescents...avoid all animal products.

Answer the following questions with a sentence:

6 What makes people overweight?
7 What is junk food? Give examples.
8 Where does dietary fibre come from?
9 What are the other effects of eating too much sugar apart from obesity?
10 What are the rules to remember when feeding convalescents?

11 Find out about the fat content of different meats and note which ones have the least. Investigate ways of making tasty and nutritious meat dishes using little fat in the cooking, and using meat with low fat content.

12 Prepare a folder to display in your home economics room to show some of the faults of modern eating habits. Call it 'Hazards of modern feeding'. Cut out pictures from magazines to illustrate your work. Include:
a your own recipe for good health,
b rules to follow to give young children good eating habits.

13 Try cooking food in a 'dry fry' pan or one with a non-stick coating. (You need less fat to stop the food sticking in these pans and the food should be less 'greasy' because it will absorb less fat.) Try cooking food in a Chinese wok or try out a recipe for Chinese 'dry fry' 'stir fry' vegetables using an ordinary pan. What advantages are there in this method of cooking?

14 An unsuitable meal for an elderly person would be:
A small piece of fried fish with batter
A large portion of chips
Steamed syrup pudding with treacle sauce
This could be improved by
a supplying a larger piece of fish cooked without batter,
b changing the chips to a small portion of potatoes boiled in their skins,
c serving stewed fruit with egg custard instead of syrup pudding and sauce.
Why would these suggestions be an improvement?

15 Compare the cost for a week of
a making bread
b buying bread
for a family of four with two adults who are both moderately active, a teenage boy and a five year old girl.

4 The food we eat

4.1 Meat

Some facts about meat

Meat is made up of **muscle** and **fat**. You can see this by pulling a small piece of meat apart using two needles and looking at it under a magnifying glass.

Muscle is made of long strands fixed together with a transparent 'skin' wrapped around. The long strands are called **fibres** and the skin is called **connective tissue**.

Fat shows as white streaks in the muscle called **marbling**. Some meat also has a layer of fat on the outside, especially if it is from an old animal.

Tough or tender?

Meat is 'tough' or 'tender' depending on what part of the animal it comes from. Meat from the parts of the animal that have the most exercise, such as the legs and neck, has tough, long muscle fibres and strong connective tissue.

Muscles from the backbone of the animal have less exercise, so this meat has shorter fibres and less connective tissue. It is more tender. Loin chops, fillet steak, rump steak and best end chops all come from these areas.

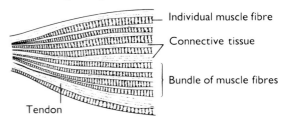

Cut lengthways

Individual muscle fibre
Connective tissue
Bundle of muscle fibres
Tendon

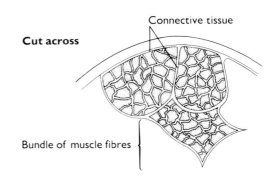

Cut across

Connective tissue
Bundle of muscle fibres

What nutrients does meat supply?

Meat is a good source of the following nutrients:

1   High quality protein — it is an excellent body building food.
2   Some fat.
3   Vitamins from the B group: thiamin, riboflavin, niacin — pork, in particular is a very good source of thiamin.
4   Iron — liver and kidney are the richest source.
5   Vitamin A — liver and kidney are very good sources of this.

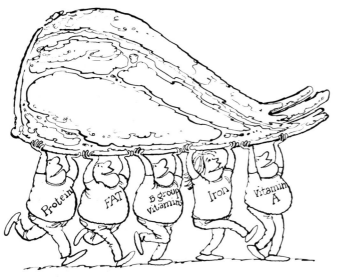

Different types of meat

It is easy to provide nutritious, interesting and varied meals with meat, because it is so versatile. The table shows the many different kinds of meat.

Meat	Animal source
Pork	Pig
Mutton Lamb	Sheep
Beef Veal	Cattle
Poultry	Chicken, Turkey, Duck
Rabbit	Rabbit
Offal	The edible part of the inside of the animal e.g. liver, heart, tongue, kidneys.

Cuts of meat

The charts show some of the cuts of meat.

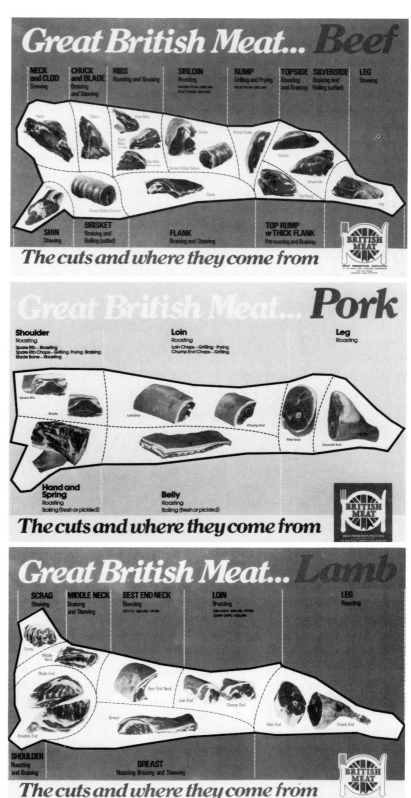

Great British Meat... Beef

NECK and CLOD	CHUCK and BLADE	RIBS	SIRLOIN	RUMP	TOPSIDE	SILVERSIDE	LEG
Stewing	Braising and Stewing	Roasting and Braising	Roasting	Grilling and Frying	Roasting and Braising	Braising and Boiling (salted)	Stewing

SHIN Stewing · **BRISKET** Braising and Boiling (salted) · **FLANK** Braising and Stewing · **TOP RUMP or THICK FLANK** Pot-roasting and Braising

The cuts and where they come from

Great British Meat... Pork

Shoulder Roasting · Spare Rib – Roasting · Spare Rib Chops – Grilling · Frying · Braising · Blade Bone – Roasting

Loin Roasting · Loin Chops – Grilling · Frying · Chump End Chops – Grilling

Leg Roasting

Hand and Spring Roasting · Boiling (fresh or pickled) · **Belly** Roasting · Boiling (fresh or pickled)

The cuts and where they come from

Great British Meat... Lamb

SCRAG	MIDDLE NECK	BEST END NECK	LOIN	LEG
Stewing	Braising and Stewing	Roasting	Roasting	Roasting

SHOULDER Roasting and Braising · **BREAST** Roasting Braising and Stewing

The cuts and where they come from

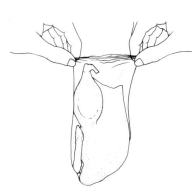

When planning meat dishes do not forget that **offal**, **chicken** and **rabbit** are good alternatives to beef, lamb and pork. They provide variety, are often cheaper and are very nutritious.

Offal

Offal includes liver, kidney, heart, sweetbreads (the glands of the thymus and pancreas from calves and lambs), tripe (the stomach lining from a calf or ox) and sheep and ox tongues.

Do not forget that liver and kidney are excellent sources of iron. Look back to page 20 to remind yourself how vitamin-C-rich food can help the body to absorb iron.

Chicken and rabbit

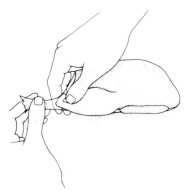

Chicken and rabbit are now quite cheap and can be made into delicious dishes for main meals. They contain plenty of easily digested protein with little fat, so they are useful for meals for slimmers, invalids or elderly people. Chicken and rabbit also have a small amount of B group vitamins, iron and phosphorus.

Freezing chicken

Chicken freezes very well and does not deteriorate if packed properly. The chicken or chicken pieces should be wrapped in heavy duty polythene, foil or freezer bags, and the air pressed from the package before sealing. The package should then be labelled and quickly frozen and stored at − 18°C. An uncooked chicken will keep for up to twelve months.

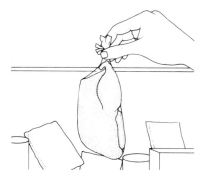

Stuffed chicken or a cooked chicken dish may be frozen in the same way, but these should not be kept for more than three months.

Always thaw the chicken thoroughly before use. You can do this in one of the following ways:

1 in a refrigerator for 24 hours, or
2 in a micro-wave oven. Use the booklet supplied with the cooker. Follow the instructions very carefully.

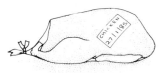

Cooking meat

Fact	Using the fact

1 There are two types of connective tissue:
  a **collagen** which can be softened by cooking,
  b **elastin** which remains tough.
	Choose meat carefully. Do not buy it if it has a lot of gristle.

2 At temperatures below 100°C, collagen slowly changes to a soft, soluble substance called **gelatin** and the meat becomes tender.	Cook cuts with lots of connective tissue in moist heat. Stewing and braising are good methods.
3 The protein in meat, which is called **myosin**, **coagulates** with heat. As the temperature increases the meat hardens and the juices with vitamins and minerals in them are squeezed out.	Do not cook any meat at too high a temperature, or it will shrink and you will lose some nutrients. Use the meat juices to make gravy.
4 Tender cuts have short, tender fibres and little connective tissue.	Chops, leg of lamb and other tender cuts can be cooked quickly using dry heat. Grilling, roasting and frying are good methods.
5 Mechanical action will break down the tissues and separate the fibres.	Mince, beat or dice cheaper cuts of meat, before cooking, to make them tender.
6 Soaking meat in **marinade** helps to break down connective tissue. Ingredients for a marinade include cider, wine, lemon juice, vinegar and special preparations using the tenderizers **papain** and **bromelin**. (Papain is extracted from the **papaya** plant and bromelin from pineapple juice.) *Special fact*: these tenderizers are based on an **enzyme** (a substance which speeds up processes) which will dissolve protein. When meat is injected with or soaked in a liquid containing pineapple juice or papain, and is left for some time, some of the protein in the meat is dissolved. This helps the meat to be more tender when cooked. Scientists call these protein dissolving enzymes **proteolytic enzymes**.	Use marinades and fruit juice to soak meat, before cooking, to tenderize it.

Shopping for meat

Before you go shopping, decide what recipe and method of cooking you are going to use. Then you can make your choice of meat. Follow these guidelines:

1. Lean meat with a coarse grain has longer and bigger bundles of muscle fibre. It should be cooked by a moist method such as braising or stewing. Slow cookers or pressure cookers are good pieces of equipment to use with this type of meat.
2. Lean meat with a smooth and velvety texture has shorter muscle fibres. It is suitable for dry, quicker methods of cooking such as frying, grilling or roasting.
3. The fat on meat should be firm and dry. There should not be too much of it on the outside of the lean.
4. Marbling (flecks of fat in the lean) is good. The fat melts into the lean during cooking. This makes the meat juicy and gives it a good flavour.
5. Colour is **not** an indication of quality in meat. Only freshly-cut meat is brightly coloured. Meat protein changes from purple to bright red and then to brown after it has been in the air for a short time.
6. On lamb, the paper-like skin that covers the fat should be soft and stretchy, not hard and wrinkled.

Choosing and identifying meat may be easier in self-service shops because it is usually labelled. Sometimes there is cooking advice on the label. Some independent butchers have attractive charts showing cuts and appropriate recipes. These too make it easier for you to recognize different cuts.

Things to do

1. *Explain what makes meat tough or tender.*
2. *What is a 'marinade'? Find some examples from cookery books.*
3. *Try out some of the recipes using a marinade in your practical class.*

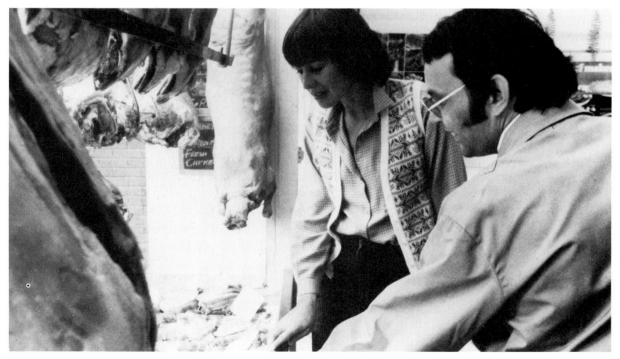

4.2 Fish

Some facts about fish

Fish is not the most economical food to buy because there is a lot of waste in the head, bones and skin or shell. However, it provides variety in the diet as well as being very nutritious. Most fish has a delicate flavour and has to be cooked and served carefully.

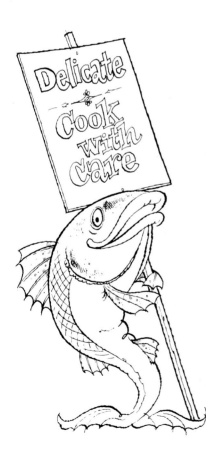

Fish and nutrients

All fish contain protein of higher biological value. Oily fish also contain fat and vitamins A and D. Canned oily fish (sardines, pilchards) contain calcium, because the bones have been softened by the canning process and may be eaten.

The livers of white fish, particularly cod and halibut, contain oil. The oil is extracted and used as a food supplement for babies and young children. The oil is a very rich source of fat and vitamins A and D.

All fish contain B group vitamins, iron and phosphorus. Sea fish is a good source of iodine and **fluorine**, which is thought to help keep tooth enamel in good condition.

Types of fish

There are two main types of fish. They are grouped according to how much fat they have in their flesh.

1   **White fish** — haddock, coley (or saithe), cod, plaice and halibut. There is no oil in the flesh of this group. The oil is in the liver in these fish.
2   **Fatty** or **oily fish** — mackerel, herring and salmon. These fish have oil in the flesh. The oil makes the flesh of these fish dark. The fat is 'invisible' fat and raises the energy value of the flesh.

There is another group of fish called **shellfish**. This includes crabs, lobsters, prawns and shrimps, which are called **crustaceans**. It also includes mussels which are **molluscs**. Shellfish are usually more expensive to buy than white or oily fish.

For many years cod has been Great Britain's favourite fish. Because of this heavy demand, it is now in short supply. Fishermen have taken so many fish from the sea that the cod cannot breed fast enough to make up their numbers. This also means that cod is becoming very expensive.

Now we need to give the fish a chance to increase their numbers. We can do this by eating other fish. **Coley** (or **saithe**) can be cooked and served in the same ways as cod, and it is a much cheaper fish to buy. You can also try dabs, flounders and witch sole, as these are both economical and plentiful.

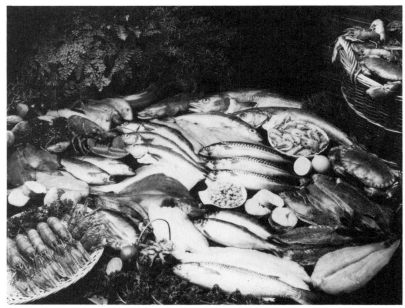

Some of the fish that can be bought in Britain

Cooking fish

Fact	Using the fact
1 Fish has little connective tissue. The little it has is all collagen.	Fish needs a shorter cooking time than meat, and a lower temperature.
2 The protein in fish will shrink if cooked too fiercely.	To prevent juices being lost, heat gently. If fish is dry because of shrinkage serve it with a sauce.

All quick methods of cooking are suitable for fish. Dry methods such as **grilling** and **frying**, with oil or fat added to prevent drying are suitable for all types of fish. Remember, however, that these methods increase the energy value of each portion.

Poaching and **steaming** are other suitable methods. These methods leave the fish moist, which is particularly good for white fish. When poaching, milk or water may be used to cook the fish, and then the liquid can be used to make a sauce.

Fish can be cooked when it is frozen. Add an extra few minutes to the cooking time, or follow the instructions on the packet. A micro-wave oven is very good for thawing and cooking fish because it keeps the moisture in the fish.

Shopping for fish

How to buy fish

There are three ways to buy fish:

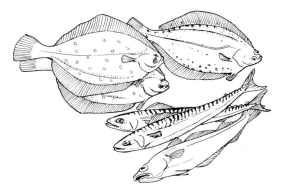

1   Whole — e.g. dabs, plaice, sole (a very expensive flat fish), small haddock, mackerel and herring. Whole fish are cheaper per kilo than fish steaks or fillets, because the fishmonger does not have to spend time boning (filleting) them.

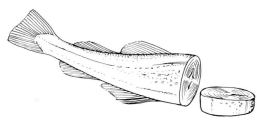

2   Steaks or cutlets — slices are cut across the fish, including a slice of the backbone. Examples are coley cutlet and haddock cutlet.

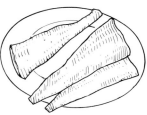

3   Fillets — here the fish is carefully removed from the bones. Haddock, coley, plaice and many other fish can be bought filleted.

Choosing fresh fish

If you are able to buy fresh fish look for the following things:

1   Bright, moist eyes — do not buy any fish with dull eyes.
2   Plenty of shiny, moist scales.
3   A fresh, 'fishy' smell.

Choosing frozen fish

A fishmonger selling fresh fish is quite a rare sight these days. However, it is possible to buy very good frozen fish. Fish are often frozen on the boats while at sea. The fish are caught, cleaned and frozen immediately, so they are really fresh. When they reach the shore, they are already frozen.

When buying frozen fish, choose a well-known brand because it is difficult to tell how good a fish is when it is frozen. Fish should be frozen quickly. If it is frozen slowly, large ice crystals form. These push the flesh of the fish out of shape. When badly frozen fish is thawed, a lot of moisture comes out. This has two results:

1   The fish may be dry when cooked.
2   Water-soluble vitamins such as the B group may be lost.

Things to do

1   *Find out what fish are found around the British Isles. Are these fish all available at your local fishmongers or supermarket?*

2   *Suggest ways of cooking other kinds of fish to take the place of cod in family meals.*

3   *Learn how to fillet fish. It is worth learning to do this because it is cheaper to buy a whole fish and then fillet it yourself.*

4.3 Eggs

Some facts about eggs

Eggs are important in providing good meals. The diagram shows the three parts of an egg.

The yolk

The **yolk** contains all the nutrients a young chick needs to grow. It contains:

Protein of higher biological value
Fat
Vitamin A, carotene (this makes the egg yolk yellow and is changed into vitamin A in the body)

It also contains small amounts of

Vitamin D
Riboflavin, thiamin
Calcium, phosphorous and iron

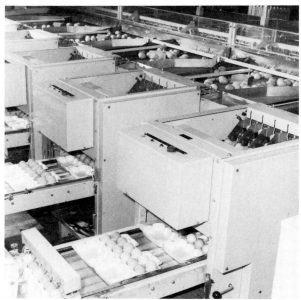

An egg packing station

The white

The **white** contains:

A lot of water
protein of higher biological value
Riboflavin

The shell

The **shell** is made from **calcium carbonate** (chalk). It protects the egg. It contains tiny holes (pores) that let air through. This means that it is **porous**. Notice the air pocket in the diagram. As the egg gets older, the air space gets bigger, because the porous shell lets air through into the egg.

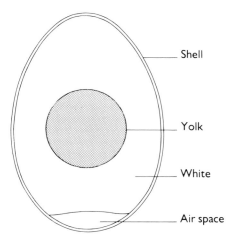

Shell

Yolk

White

Air space

Special fact
There is no difference nutritionally between white and brown eggs, or between light and dark coloured yolks. The colour of the shell and the yolk vary according to the breed of the hen and what it has eaten.

Storing eggs

The contents of an egg shrink when it is kept for a long time, because the moisture inside can get out through the holes in the shell. Bacteria can also get in through the holes. The bacteria use the air and the sulphur in the egg protein to make a gas called **hydrogen sulphide**. This is what gives a 'rotten egg' smell.

Eggs should be stored *cool* and *dry* with the *round* end up. Because the shell is porous, keep eggs away from strong-smelling food.

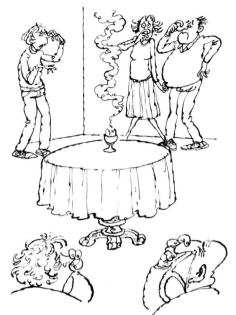

How fresh is an egg?

You can test an egg for freshness yourself. To do this make up a solution of 300 ml of water with 25 g of salt. Put it in a tall jar or jug. Place an egg carefully in the solution. Notice what happens. Did the egg float? If it did, can you explain why?

The air space in an old egg is bigger than in a new one. This makes the egg more buoyant (it floats easier because it is lighter). Try the test again, with an egg you know is really fresh, and with one you know is older and see what happens.

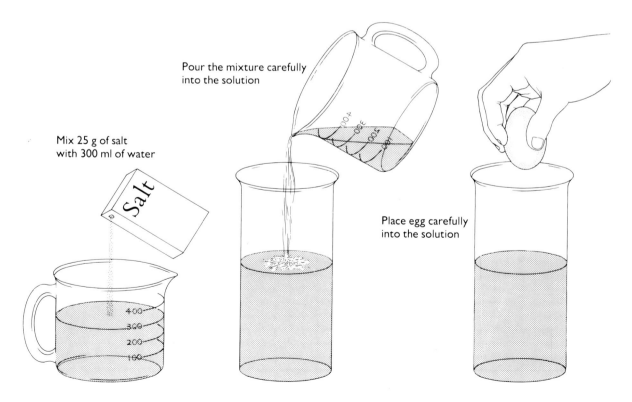

Pour the mixture carefully into the solution

Mix 25 g of salt with 300 ml of water

Place egg carefully into the solution

Cooking with eggs

Fact	Using the fact

1 Eggs protein coagulates with heat; the white at 60°C, the yolk at 68°C (a higher temperature because of the fat in the yolk) and the whole egg at 64°C. 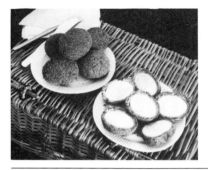	Eggs can be boiled or poached in boiling water. the water should be boiling gently not vigorously. Adding **vinegar** to water for poaching eggs raises the temperature of the water. This speeds up coagulation so that the egg keeps it shape.
	
	    Eggs can be fried gently in oil or fat. This gives very quick coagulation. Frying in very hot fat can make the egg leathery.
	
	    Eggs can be used for **coating** food with breadcrumbs, as on Scotch eggs. The egg coagulates quickly and holds the crumbs onto the outside. This stops the oil from soaking into the food and makes a crisp coating.
	
	    Binding — egg is added to mixtures to hold ingredients together, as in fish cakes.
	
	    Clearing — white of egg and the crushed shell may be added to soups and homemade jellies. The egg coagulates when it is heated and all the 'bits are attracted to it. They can then be taken out by straining, leaving the liquid clear and sparkling. This is called **clarifying**.

2 When egg is heated with a liquid, the protein can enclose tiny particles of the liquid when it coagulates. This makes the mixture thicken.
 	
    As the temperature increases, the protein becomes harder and squeezes the liquid out. This causes **curdling**.
	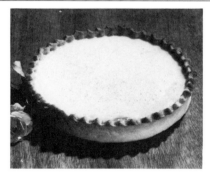 When eggs are combined with milk and then heated, they thicken the mixture. Egg custards are a good example of this.
	
	    This can happen with egg custards. Heat gently and use a water-bath to prevent curdling. The water in the water-bath **insulates** the mixture from too much heat.

3 When egg white is beaten, the protein partly coagulates. Air is added to the mixture by beating. The air bubbles are surrounded by thin, set egg white and a foam is made.	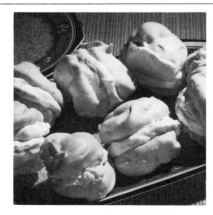 Beaten egg whites can be used to put air into a mixture. The air expands (gets bigger) when it is in the oven and the mixture rises. Meringues are made in this way. Cakes are another example, particularly whisked and creamed mixtures.

Buying eggs

Grade	Description
A	Fresh eggs, naturally clean, shell intact, internally perfect. The air pocket must not be bigger than 6 mm.
B	Downgraded because of e.g. blood spots, or because the eggs have been preserved in some way. The air pocket must not be bigger than 9 mm.
C	For manufacturing use only — not on sale to the public.

EEC egg grades

Size	Weight
1	70 g and over
2	65-70 g
3	60-65 g
4	55-60 g
5	50-55 g
6	45-50 g
7	under 45 g

EEC egg sizes

In the EEC (European Economic Community), eggs are graded and priced by weight and quality. There are three quality grades and seven size grades as you can see in the tables.

When you buy eggs in the shops, you will find these size and grade 'codes' on the box. You will also find a set of three numbers. The first number tells you which EEC country the eggs were packed in. The table shows you what these are.

The second number tells you the region of the country and the last number tells you the licence number of the packing station which packed the eggs. The drawing shows you what these codes look like.

No.	Country
1	Belgium
2	W Germany
3	France
4	Italy
5	Luxembourg
6	The Netherlands
7	Denmark
8	Ireland
9	UK
10	Greece

EEC codes for countries

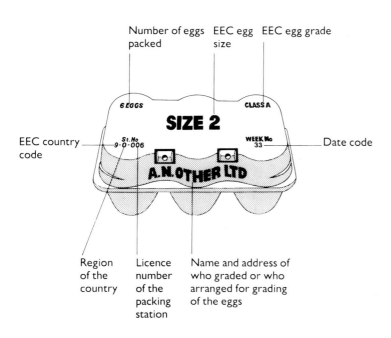

Number of eggs packed · EEC egg size · EEC egg grade

6 EGGS · CLASS A

SIZE 2

EEC country code — St. No 9·0·006 · WEEK No 33 — Date code

A. N. OTHER LTD

Region of the country · Licence number of the packing station · Name and address of who graded or who arranged for grading of the eggs

Things to do

1 *Make a list of dishes which show the part eggs can play in the family diet.*

2 *Choose one way of cooking a whole egg to make a dish for breakfast. From what you have learned, say what special care has to be taken during the cooking and explain why.*

3 *Break the code on a box of eggs.*

4.4 **Milk**

Some facts about milk

Milk is nine-tenths water. It is sometimes called the perfect food, but this is not strictly true. It is a rich source of protein of higher biological value and calcium, phosphorus, vitamin A and riboflavin. It also has small amounts of vitamin C, vitamin D and thiamin. But, it is not a high energy food. The cream that comes to the top of the milk is the fat. The slightly sweet taste of milk comes from **lactose**, a sugar.

Milk contains some **bacteria** which change the lactose into a sour-tasting substance called **lactic acid**. This acid makes the protein (called casein) in milk turn into a solid or **curd**. So you get sour, curdled milk. This tends to happen if milk is added to mixtures which are **acidic** or if milk is kept in a warm place.

Try this experiment to see for yourself: Prepare two basins with equal, small quantities of milk in each. To one add 1 tablespoon of vinegar. To the other add 1 tablespoon of lemon juice. (Both vinegar and lemon juice are *acidic* – sour tasting.)

What happens to the milk in each case? Make a note of what you see.

Now repeat the experiment, but this time use hot milk in each basin.

Does anything different happen?

You need to be very careful when making dishes which include milk and acidic substances. For example, when making tomato soup you need to watch that the juice from the tomatoes does not curdle the milk. You can do this by adding flour to thicken the soup.

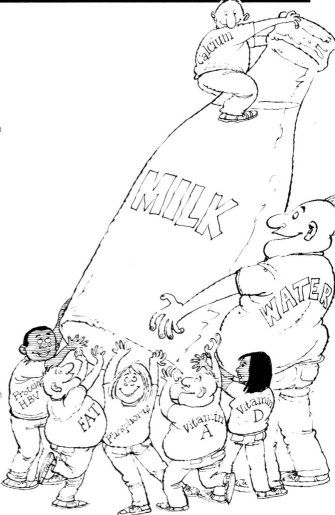

Digesting milk

Milk is very easy to digest. This makes it a particularly valuable food for invalids, children and the elderly. The protein in milk is coagulated into a hard clot by **rennin** which is in the stomach.

You can see how this happens by making **junket**. This is a nutritious and easily digested pudding.

Junket is made by warming milk to blood heat (above 36°C) and then adding a few drops of **rennet** (a commercially prepared liquid containing rennin). The clot forms as the junket cools.

Find out whether the clot formed is **acid** or **alkaline**. Do this by putting a few drops of litmus solution on the clot. The solution will turn red if the clot is acidic and blue if it is alkaline.

Burn a little of the clot on an enamel plate or tray and note the smell. Proteins smell like singed hair when burnt.

What does the burning clot smell of? Do you think there is protein in it?

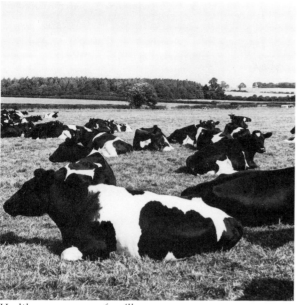
Healthy cows mean safe milk

Different types of milk

Milk is an ideal place for bacteria to grow because it is so rich in nutrients. This means that we need to make sure that the milk people get is safe to use. This is done by:

1 Creating herds of cows that are clean and healthy — milk-giving herds are checked carefully regularly, and all milk sold is from **TT (Tuberculin Tested)** or **Accredited** herds, that is from herds which are healthy.
2 Treating the milk in various ways before it is packaged for sale — most of the treatment is heat treatment.

The table shows the types of milk available.

Name	Bottle top	How it has been treated	How long it will keep
Pasteurized	Silver	Heated to 72°C for at least 15 seconds and cooled rapidly. The treatment destroys some of the thiamin and vitamin C. Taste is hardly altered.	1-3 days in a cool place. At least 3 days in a refrigerator.
Homogenized	Red	Milk is spun in machines to distribute fat evenly through it. There is no cream on top. Taste is slightly altered.	1-3 days in a cool place. At least 3 days in a refrigerator.
Channel Islands and South Devon	Gold	Creamier milk from Jersey, Guernsey and South Devon breeds (contains more fat and fat-soluble vitamins).	1-3 days in a cool place. At least 3 days in a refrigerator.
Sterilized	Crown cap	Homogenized milk heated to a higher temperature than for pasteurization. It has a 'cooked' taste. Much thiamin is destroyed.	Keeps unopened for several days without a refrigerator.
Ultra-high temperature (UHT) or 'long-life' milk	Foil-lined container	Homogenized milk heated to a high temperature (135°-150°C) for 1-3 seconds. The taste is slightly altered. UHT milk has the same food value as pasteurized milk.	Keeps for several months in a *cool* place if *unopened*. When opened, treat as fresh milk. NB it is usually date-stamped.

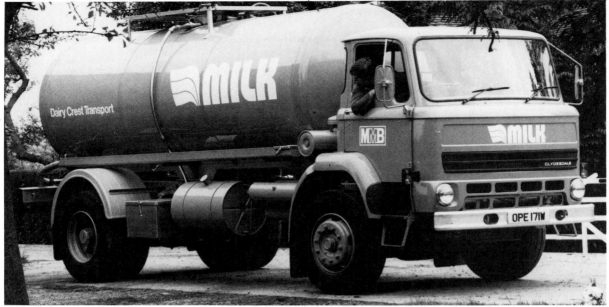
Transporting milk

Storing milk

Milk sours more quickly when it is warm, so store milk in a *cool* place. Milk should always be stored *covered* in *clean* containers.

If milk is left on the doorstep for any length of time, particularly in the sun, most of the vitamin C and riboflavin will be destroyed. Try and take milk inside as soon as it is delivered. If milk is heated for too long the thiamin will be destroyed, so heat milk gently and for a short time.

Milk and transport

Because milk is nine-tenths water, it is bulky and expensive to transport. Some methods of pocessing reduce that bulk and make transporting easier and cheaper.

One way is to remove the water by **evaporation** and produce **evaporated milk**. This contains about 25% less water than fresh milk. It is sealed in cans and has a long 'shelf life' if unopened. This makes it useful as an emergency stand-by. If sugar is added it becomes sweetened **condensed milk**, another useful stand-by.

Milk may be **dried** by removing all the water. There are many different kinds of dried milk available and they are all good ways of keeping milk in **concentrated** form. Some of them have the fat

removed. These are labelled 'dried skimmed milk'. They are useful if you are trying to reduce the fat content of a meal.

Freezing milk

UHT (long-life) milk and dried milk keep so well that there is no need to freeze milk for emergencies. If milk is frozen, it should be in cartons and not in a bottle. The milk will expand as it freezes and crack the bottle.

Things to do

1 *Compare the **unit price** of the various tinned and dried milks available. The 'unit price' is the amount it costs to make a pint of milk from each product. How do these prices compare with the cost of a pint of fresh milk?*

2 *Use tinned or dried milk instead of fresh milk in a recipe e.g. a blancmange or milk pudding. Taste the dish. How does it differ from the dish made with fresh milk? Make notes about your results.*

3 *Study the list of ingredients on different dried or tinned milks. Do they all contain the same nutrients? Notice particularly the ingredients in dried milk for babies.*

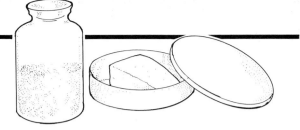

4.5 Cheese

Facts about cheese

It takes one pint of milk to make 60 g of cheese. This means cheese is a very rich and concentrated source of most of the nutrients milk contains. Cheese is an excellent source of protein, calcium, fat and vitamin A and it also contains riboflavin. However, cheese does not contain sugar, because the lactose in the milk is changed to lactic acid when it is made into cheese.

Cheese is a useful food for a number of reasons:

1. It is high in nutritive value.
2. It can be used in a number of ways and can provide variety in the diet.
3. It is easy to store and takes up little space.
4. It is useful for emergencies.
5. It is available in many forms and flavours.
6. Tasty meals can be easily made from it.
7. It is quite inexpensive.

Buying and storing cheese

1. Firm cheese, such as cheddar, will keep longer than soft cheese, so you can buy it in larger quantities.
2. Because soft cheese does not keep so long, buy only enough for your immediate needs.
3. Store cheese in a box or polythene wrapper in a cool place. The refrigerator may dry cheese, but you can prevent this by wrapping it well.
4. Store grated cheese ready for use in a glass jar and keep it in a cool, dry place.
5. If cheese is served too cold, it loses some of its flavour. Take cheese from the refrigerator some time before serving.

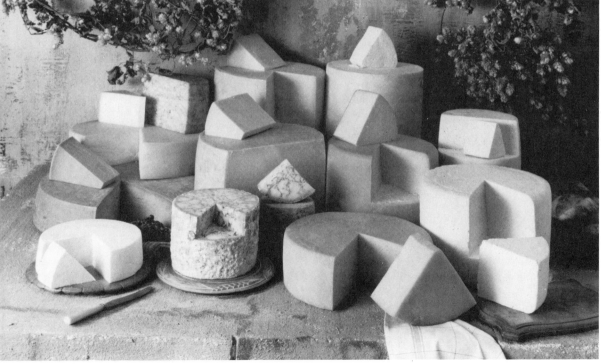

Some of the cheese made in Britain

Cooking with cheese

Fact	Using the fact
1 When cheese is heated the fat melts and separates.	It is better to grate cheese before cooking and mix it with a starchy ingredient which will absorb the fat. This makes it nicer to at and easier to digest.
2 High temperatures make the cheese protein coagulate quickly. This makes the cheese tough, stringy and elastic. Then it will not blend easily with other ingredients. It may make it difficult to digest.	Cook for a short time at a low temperature. In this way the cheese will blend easily with other ingredients.

Because cheese is so concentrated, you need only a little at a time. Some cheeses e.g. Brie and Cheddar have a high fat content. This should be taken into account when planning meals. Cheeses like Edam and cottage cheese which are labelled as 'low fat' may be a better choice than the high fat types. It is a useful food to include in quick lunches or packed meals, when you do not have much space. Remember that cheese is more difficult to digest than milk. It should be cooked and served with care.

Things to do

1 *There is not enough room in this book to describe all the different cheeses. Make your own study of the different types. You will find books to help you in the library.*

2 *Why is cheese thought to be:*
   a *a good snack,*
   b *a good alternative to meat and fish,*
   c *a concentrated food,*
   d *a party food?*

3 *Make a list of as many types of cheeses as you can. Find out the proportion of fat in each one.*

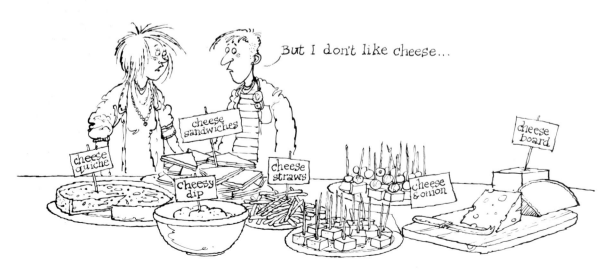

But I don't like cheese...

cheese quiche — cheese sandwiches — Cheesy dip — cheese straws — cheese & onion — cheese board

4.6 **Fruit**

Some facts about fruit

The food value of fruit varies. Blackcurrants are an excellent source of vitamin C, but citrus fruits probably contribute more vitamin C to our diet than any other food because we eat more of them. Oranges, peaches and apricots supply some carotene. Oranges, strawberries, cantaloupe melon and dried fruits such as figs, dates, prunes and apricots are all good sources of iron and calcium.

The carbohydrates (sugars and starches) in fruit are **sugar** and **cellulose**. Ripe fruits contain more sugar than unripe ones. The skin and pulp of fruits contain cellulose. This fibrous material cannot be digested by the body. Instead it helps to give bulk and moisture to the waste material our bodies have to get rid of and so it prevents bowel disorders.

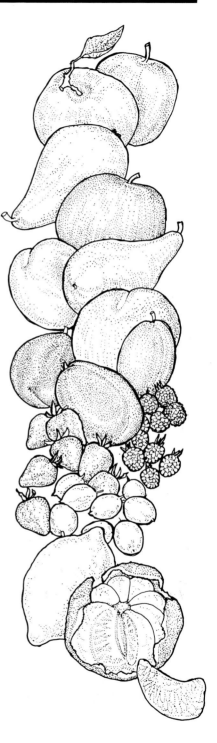

Types of fruit

Fruits can be grouped into:

1   **Hard fruit** e.g. apples and pears.
2   **Soft fruit** e.g. strawberries, raspberries, plums, peaches, apricots and gooseberries.
3   **Citrus fruits** e.g. oranges, grapefruits, lemon and limes.

Storing fruit

Ripe fruits are **perishable** and are best stored in a cool place. The vegetable drawer of a refrigerator is a good place because it stops the fruit drying out.

Berries should not be washed before storing, as this makes them more likely to spoil. Bananas should never be stored in a refrigerator. Strong smelling fruit such as melon and pineapple must be covered before they are put in the refrigerator.

Frozen fruit (which has been bought already frozen) should not be allowed to thaw before it is stored in the freezer.

Canned fruit will keep for a long time if it is left unopened in a cool, dry, place. Once it is opened it becomes perishable.

Dried fruit should be kept closely wrapped in a cool, dry place. When reconstituted (mixed with water) and cooked the fruit becomes perishable.

Preparing and serving fruit

One of the great advantages of fruit is that it can be eaten raw. This **conserves** much of the vitamin C present. When the fruit has to be prepared or peeled, remember that vitamin C is most concentrated just under the skin. Either

1 peel thinly, or
2 eat unpeeled fruit.

Fruit also looks more attractive if it is unpeeled. For example, unpeeled red apples give a lot of colour to a salad.

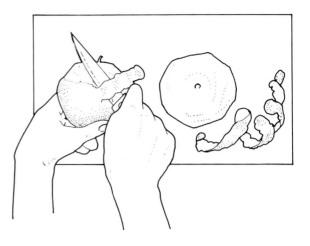

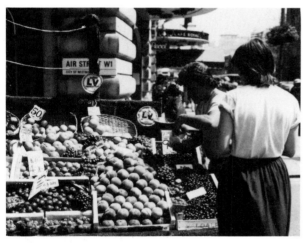

Buying fruit

The price of fruit is not always a sign of quality. Fruit in season is generally cheaper and better quality than fruit out of season.

Good quality fruit is free from bruises, moulds and blemishes. Most types of fruit should be firm, and hard fruit should be crisp. So look for fruit that is **sound** and **crisp** or **firm**.

Fruit and convenience

Ready-prepared fruit is available in many forms. It can be canned, frozen or dried. This not only saves time and energy but means that fruit is available out of season. You will find out more about these 'convenience' fruits in Unit 6.

Things to do

1 *Calculate the cost of one portion of fresh fruit and compare it with the cost of the same fruit canned, frozen or dried.*

2 *Make a list of the ways fruit can be stored.*

3 *Suggest ways of including fruit in main meals.*

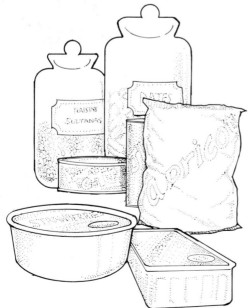

4.7 Vegetables

Some facts about vegetables

The nutritive value of vegetables varies from type to type, but they all contain water and cellulose. This makes them a good source of dietary fibre.

Soya beans supply protein of higher biological value. Other beans and peas supply protein of lower biological value as well as iron and some vitamin B. Red and green peppers, raw cabbage, sprouts, kale spinach, cauliflower, broccoli and peas are good sources of vitamin C.

Potatoes contribute a high proportion of the vitamin C in most people's diet, not because they contain a lot of the vitamin , but because people eat a lot of them. New potatoes contain more vitamin C than old ones. Carrots, spinach and other green and orange vegetables are good sources of carotene.

Most of the root and tuber vegetables contain starch. Green leaf vegetables contain some calcium and iron.

Types of vegetables

Vegetables are grouped according to which part of the plant is eaten.

Leaves — cabbage, spinach, sprouts, endive and kale.
Stems — celery and asparagus.
Flowers — cauliflower, broccoli and calabrese.
Fruits — red and green peppers, cucumber and tomatoes.
Roots — carrots, parsnips, beetroot and radishes.
Tubers — potatoes.
Bulbs — onions.
Legumes (seeds) — peas and beans.

Storing vegetables

Green vegetables and salad plants are best eaten soon after you buy them. If they have to be stored put them into the salad drawer of the refrigerator. They will keep fresh in a covered dish or saucepan for a short time.

Root vegetables are best kept in a rack in a cool, dry, well-ventilated place.

Cooking vegetables

Turn back to page 17 to remind yourself how to avoid losing vitamin C when cooking vegetables. Remember that vitamin C is water-soluble and so it is best to eat vegetables like cabbage and carrots raw.

Some vegetables, however, cannot be eaten raw. They have to be cooked to soften the cellulose and cook the starch. During cooking, the starch absorbs water, swells and becomes softer. Vegetables also change in colour and flavour when they are cooked.

An important point to remember is that careful cooking protects the colour, flavour, texture and nutritive value of vegetables.

Buying vegetables

Freshly picked vegetables have the best flavour and food value. So it is a good idea to grow your own if you can.

Storage destroys vitamin C, so choose fresh vegetables. These should be firm and crisp with a good colour. Reject vegetables with wilted leaves or shrivelled skin. Small to medium-sized vegetables are usually best value for money. Large ones tend to be tough and 'woody' because they are old.

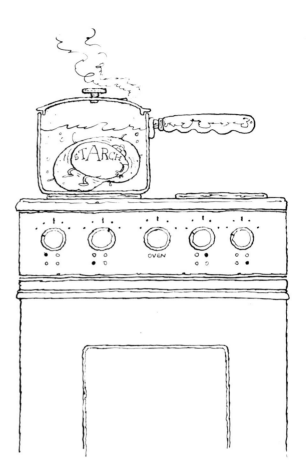

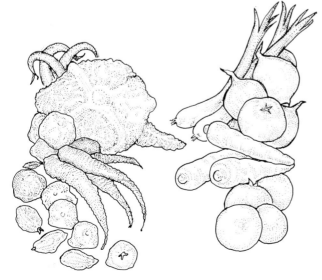

Things to do

1 *Next time you prepare potatoes, taste a little piece raw. Compare it with the taste of a cooked potato. Do you think there is a change in taste during cooking?*

2 *Dip a small piece of raw potato in **iodine** and note any change of colour. If the potato turns blue-black this means that it contains starch. This is the starch that absorbs the water when potatoes are boiled.*

3 *Write down how you can save vitamin C when cooking vegetables.*

4.8 Cereals

Facts about cereals

Cereals are cultivated grasses. From the beginning of civilization people have harvested all types of cereals for food. Cereals include wheat, rice, oats, rye, maize and barley.

Cereals form the basis of many meals all over the world. They are often called **staple foods**. Wheat is basic to the diets of people in Europe, America, Australia and some parts of Asia. Rice is the basis of meals in the Far East and India. Generally the cereal which grows best in a country's climate and soil is the one eaten most in that country.

Cereals are valuable because:

1 they have good keeping quality,
2 they are nutritious,
3 they are relatively cheap to grow.

In some underdeveloped countries, as much as 80% of the food eaten is supplied by one cereal. If the harvest is poor some people may die from starvation.

The cereal grain

We eat the **grain** of cereal. The plant makes this part to reproduce itself. It is like the seeds of a flowering plant. Each grain has three parts: bran, endosperm, and germ.

The **bran** is the outside covering (or husk) and has a number of layers. The **endosperm** is the white inner portion. The **germ** is at one end. It is where the new plant sprouts.

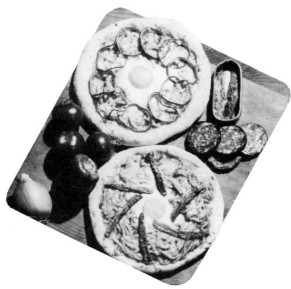

A meal based on wheat

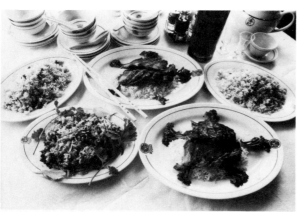

A meal based on rice

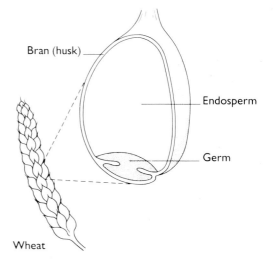

Bran (husk)

Endosperm

Germ

Wheat

Cereals and nutrients

Different parts of cereals contain different nutrients. The bran and germ contain vitamins of the B group (thiamin, riboflavin, nicotinic acid), calcium, iron and cellulose. The germ contains fat. The endosperm contains starch.

Cereals also contain protein. The protein is of lower biological value, because it does not contain all the essential amino acids, but it is still an important part of the daily protein intake. It can be supplemented with HBV protein food or other lower biological value protein foods (see pages 7 and 8). Examples of this are breakfast cereals served with milk, rice pudding and vegetable pie with pastry.

Changing cereals into food

Cereals are not usually eaten as 'whole grains'. They are refined to make them easier and more attractive to eat and more convenient to use. This can remove some of their food value.

Wheat is the main staple food for most people in the western world. It is **milled** to make flour. To make white flour the bran and the germ are removed. They make up 30% of the whole grain. (They are then used as animal feed.)

This sort of flour is described as **70% extraction**. The bran and the germ contain calcium, iron and the B group vitamins so these are lost when the bran and germ are removed. By law, white flour has to be fortified with these vitamins and minerals during manufacture.

Wholemeal flour is made from almost the whole of the grain. As a result more B group vitamins, calcium and iron remain in it after manufacture. Unfortunately, it also contains phytic acid. This can prevent iron and calcium from being absorbed for use by the body. Wholemeal flour is a better source of dietary fibre than white flour.

Rice is the main or **staple** food of nearly half the population of the world. Rice has less protein and more starch than wheat. When **brown rice** is made only the outer husk is removed so thiamin, calcium and iron are not lost.

However, when **white rice** is made these nutrients are lost because the grain is 'polished' to remove the whole of the outer casing that contains them.

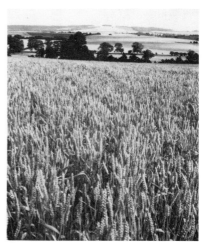

Growing wheat

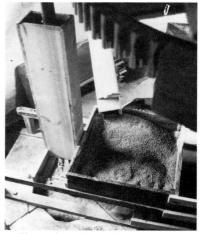

Milling wheat the old-fashioned way — in a windmill!

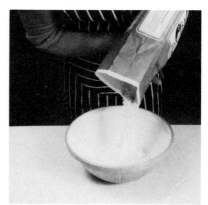

White flour

Types of cereals

Some uses of cereals

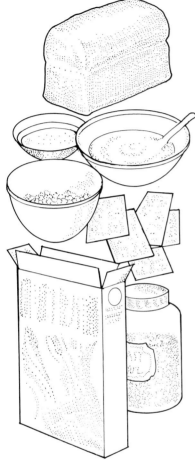

Cereal	Food	Used in cooking:	Manufactured into:
Wheat	Flour	Bread, pastry, cakes, biscuits	Bread, macaroni, spaghetti, puffed wheat, shredded wheat, semolina
Barley	Pearl barley	Soups, stews	Malt, barley water
Oats	Oatmeal	Parkin, porridge, flapjack	Oat crunchies and other breakfast cereals
Rye	Rye flour	Rye bread	'Ryvita' and some other crispbreads
Maize	Maize flour	Corn on the cob	Cornflakes, cornflour, custard and blancmange powders
Rice	Rice flour, ground rice, brown and white rice grains	Rice pudding, pilaf (pilau), risotto	Rice crispies

Breakfast cereals

There is an endless variety of ready-to-eat cereals. They are cooked and then rolled, flaked, puffed or shredded and are often made from maize, oats, wheat and rice. Some of the valuable nutrients in the grain are lost when breakfast cereals are processed. So cereals are often fortified.

Pasta

Pasta is made from **durum wheat**. It can be bought in many shapes and sizes including bows, tubes and twists. Different types are spaghetti, macaroni, vermicelli, noodles and lasagne.

Pasta is useful:

1   To extend more expensive protein food (make it go further), as in lasagne, chicken noodle soup, cannelloni and macaroni cheese.
2   As an accompaniment to meat instead of potatoes, as in chicken supreme with noodles.
3   As an ingredient in a main dish, soup or salad.

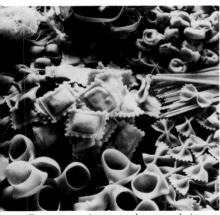

Pasta comes in many shapes and sizes

Using cereals and cereal products

Cereals are not only served with milk at breakfast time. They can also be used:

1 As a topping for casseroles or stewed fruit.
2 Crushed to make a coating for meat or fish.
3 As a biscuit base for flans and cheesecakes.
4 In cake or biscuit mixtures.

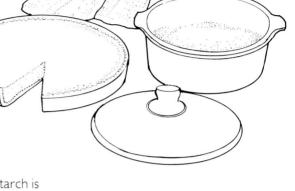

Cereals can also be cooked. This is done:

1 to improve their flavour,
2 to soften the cellulose and make the cereal edible,
3 to gelatinize the starch,
4 to produce a smooth thickened mixture (no lumps).

Cereals have a large proportion of starch. When the starch is heated it absorbs water and swells making the mixture thicken. This is called **gelatinization**. When cooking cereals you need to stop lumps from forming as the gelatinization takes place. To avoid lumps:

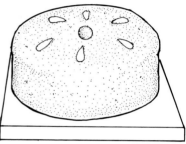

1 Cereals in large grains or pieces, such as rice and pasta, should be added to rapidly boiling water and stirred in.
2 Finer cereals, such as cornflour and flour, should be blended with small amounts of *cold* water before hot liquid is added, and stirred all the time until the mixture boils.

Things to do

1 *List the cereal products you ate yesterday. What proportion of your total food intake came from cereals?*

2 *Cook 25 g of any pasta. Weigh it after cooking. Does it weigh the same as the uncooked pasta? If not, why do you think it is different? Use the cooked pasta to make a savoury dish suitable for a main meal for yourself.*

3 *Visit the supermarket and notice the kind of cereals and cereal products offered for sale. What information is printed on the labels?*

4 *Do a 'value for money' exercise. Compare the costs and weights of different sized packets of the same breakfast cereal. Does the biggest size always provide the cheapest portion?*

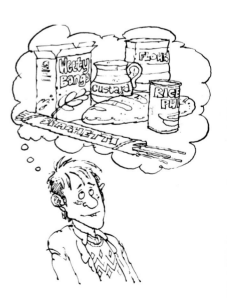

Recap 4

Fill in the blanks in the following sentences:

1   Meat is made up of _____ and _____.
2   Fish is a good source of _____.
3   Eating fruit raw _____ the vitamin C.
4   Soya beans contain protein of _____ value.
5   The edible part of cereals is the _____.

Answer the following questions:

6   Why is some meat tough and some meat tender?
7   What are the three ways of buying fish?
8   Egg shells are porous. What does this mean?
9   How should milk be stored?
10 Why is cheese a useful food? Give as many reasons as you can.

11 Compare the prices of the amount of egg, milk, fish, meat and cheese needed for one person for a main meal. Which is the best value for money? Make up a dish using this for open day. Make a chart to show your findings about different costs.

12 Examine and use a jar or can of fruit pie filling. Compare it with some fresh fruit suitable for putting in a pie. Think about the following points:
Ease of preparation...time needed for preparation...taste...texture...colour...cost. What ingredients are listed on the label of the pie filling? Is fruit mentioned? Are there any times you would use the pie filling rather than fresh fruit when making a pie?

13 Why do you think we are being encouraged to eat more fruit, vegetables and cereal products in the 1980s? Give reasons.

5 Cooking

5.1 Food and cooking

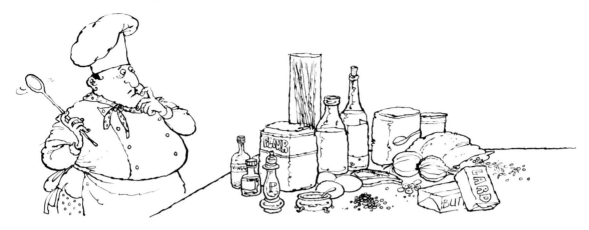

Why we cook food

1 Cooking improves the **taste**, **smell** and **appearance** of most foods.
2 It also makes some foods such as meat, easier to **chew** and **digest**.
3 Food **keeps better** and is safer to eat after cooking because the yeasts, moulds and bacteria which spoil food are destroyed.
4 **New flavours** and **colours** are sometimes made during cooking.

Cooking in moist heat

Boiling, stewing, simmering, steaming and pressure cooking are all methods of cooking by moist heat.

This is what happens to the food:

1 **Proteins** coagulate. Connective tissue of 'tough' meat (collagen) is changed to gelatin and becomes tender.
2 The **cellulose walls** of fruits and vegetables soften and break down.
3 **Starch** grains swell and absorb liquid to become jelly-like. This happens when a sauce thickens.
4 Most **minerals** and the water-soluble **vitamins** (B group and C) 'leak' into the water. Use the water for gravies, stocks and soup.
5 **Fats** melt.

No water is lost in this form of cooking. Some foods, such as rice, absorb part of the cooking liquid.

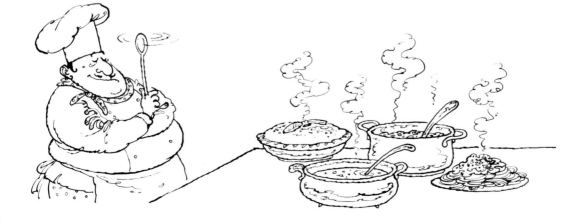

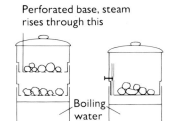

Perforated base, steam
rises through this

Boiling
water

Special pans for
steaming

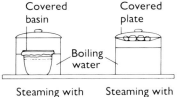

Covered
basin

Covered
plate

Boiling
water

Steaming with
a basin in
boiling water

Steaming with
a covered
plate over
boiling water

Steaming

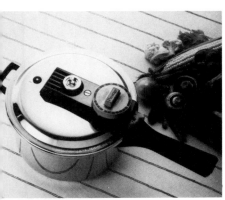

A pressure cooker

Boiling and simmering

The hot liquid used in moist heat methods passes heat to the food very quickly. It tells you on page 85 how this happens. The water can be **boiling** (for boiling vegetables) or **simmering** (near but below boiling point) when stewing and poaching.

'Boil in the bag' cooking uses boiling water indirectly: the food is sealed in the bag. Nutrients and flavour are not lost because the food is not in direct contact with the water.

Boil in the bag cooking

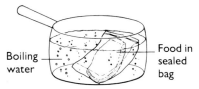

Boiling
water

Food in
sealed
bag

Steaming and pressure cooking

In **steaming** the food is cooked by the steam from boiling water. The food is not placed in the water, but in the steam above. This is a slow method of cooking, but fewer nutrients are lost.

Pressure cooking is a much quicker method of cooking food in steam. The pressure cooker is a pan with a lid which can be locked on. Food is put into the pan with a small amount of water. The water is heated until it boils, with the lid locked on. As the water boils, the pressure inside the saucepan increases. Increasing the pressure makes the water boil at a higher temperature. This means the food is cooked more quickly — in fact, it takes between a quarter and a third of the normal cooking time.

The amount of pressure is varied by putting weights on the lid. This is what happens:

At normal atmospheric pressure (15 lb per square inch or 1.05 kg per cm^2) water boils at 100°C.

If the pressure is increased by:

1   5 lb per square inch (0.35 kg per cm^2) water boils at about 107°C.
2   10 lb per square inch (0.7 kg per cm^2) water boils at about 112°C.
3   15 lb per square inch (1.05 kg per cm^2) water boils at about 120°C.

Pressure cooking is quick and cheap (because less fuel is used). It is good for making tough meat tender in a short time. More than one food can be cooked at the same time using the separators which are supplied with the pressure cooker.

Cooking in dry heat

When food is cooked by dry heat, water is driven off and the food becomes crisp. Dry heat methods of cooking are roasting, baking, grilling and frying. These cooking methods use higher temperatures than moist heat methods. This is what happens to the food:

1 **Proteins** coagulate and can harden. If meat has a lot of connective tissue, the high temperature used in dry heat cooking will harden it and make it tough and chewy.
2 **Protein and starch** combinations, such as egg glaze on bread rolls, go brown.
3 **Starch** changes colour when it is toasted or baked, to make a brown crust. **Dextrin** is the brown substance. Sugar goes yellowy-gold and eventually turns to caramel.
4 **Minerals** usually don't change at all.
5 Some **B group vitamins** and **vitamin C** are lost because of the high temperature. Fat-soluble **vitamins A** and **D** go into the melted fat.
6 **Air** and **gases** in bread and cakes expand (get bigger), so food becomes lighter and has a more 'open' texture.
7 **Fats** melt. When foods like potatoes are cooked in fat, they absorb some of the fat.

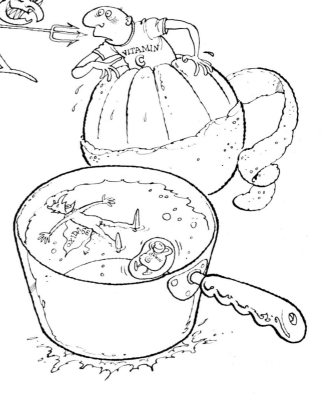

Saving vitamin C

Vitamin C is very easily destroyed by heat. It can be saved if you store, prepare and cook vitamin-C-rich food very carefully. Look at the table (pages 14 to 15) to remind you which foods have vitamin C in them.

The main sources of vitamin C are vegetables and fruit, but fruit and vegetables also have a substance in them which will destroy the vitamin. This substance is an enzyme called **oxidase**. When fruit and vegetables are peeled, chopped, shredded or crushed, the oxidase is set free and destroys the vitamin. However, if you put the food into boiling water immediately, this kills the enzyme and more of the vitamin C is saved. Other ways of saving the vitamin C in food are in the table opposite.

76

How to stop vitamin C from being destroyed

	Fact	Using the fact
1	Oxygen in air 'robs' food of vitamin C.	Store food in a cool, dark place, such as a plastic container with a tight lid in the refrigerator.
2	The enzyme oxidase is set free when food is peeled or chopped.	Do not cut and shred vitamin-C-rich foods very much. Just cut them enough to shorten the cooking time. Put the foods into boiling water immediately. Eat foods rich in vitamin C (such as cabbage) raw if possible. Use a very sharp knife for cutting them. Cook potatoes in their skins. If you peel fruit and vegetables, do it very thinly because a lot of the vitamin C is just under the skin.
3	Vitamin C is water-soluble.	Prepare and cook vegetables just before the meal is served. Do not soak the food. Cook it in a very small amount of water. Cover the pan with a lid so that you can use less water and keep air out. Cook the food for as short a time as possible and eat it as soon as it is cooked.
4	Vitamin C is 'protected' by acid.	Toss a salad in a vinegar or lemon juice dressing immediately after making it.
5	Using tinned and enamel utensils increases the loss of vitamin C.	Use plastic, nylon or stainless steel graters and strainers, and stainless steel knives for cutting vitamin-C-rich foods.

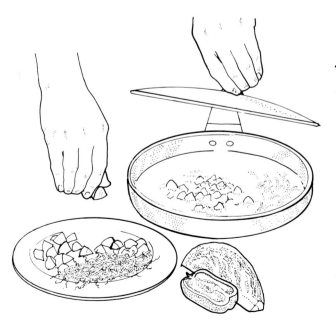

Things to do

1   *Prepare some vitamin-C-rich vegetables (like bean sprouts, cabbage and green peppers). Cut them into small pieces and immediately fry them in a little oil in a covered pan for three to five minutes. Shake the pan occasionally to stop them sticking. Serve immediately. This is a favourite Chinese way of cooking vegetables. It saves much of the vitamin C and vegetables taste good. In recipe books this is sometimes called **stir-frying**.*

2   *Design a poster to show why we cook food. Call it 'Why do we cook food?' Make sure you include the four reasons given on page 74.*

5.2 Raising agents

What are raising agents?

Raising agents are substances which make mixtures light with a 'risen' shape and open texture. They do this by making the mixtures 'rise'.

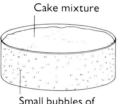

Cake mixture

Small bubbles of
air and gas

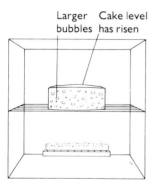

Larger   Cake level
bubbles has risen

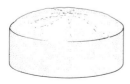

Finished cake — the gas
has now gone

The usual raising agents are **air, steam** and **carbon dioxide**. Air and steam are **physical** raising agents because they occur naturally and don't have to be made.

Carbon dioxide does have to be made. This is done by using:

1 **Bicarbonate of soda** — this is a chemical raising agent.
2 **Yeast**

Raising agents make mixtures rise because:

1 air and gas **expand** (take up more space) on heating,
2 steam has a **greater volume** (is bigger) than the liquid it comes from.

Physical or mechanical raising agents

You can put air into mixtures by sifting, rubbing in, creaming, folding, whisking and beating. Where air is being used to help a mixture rise, take great care not to let it out of the mixture once it has been put in. For example, when you make a whisked sponge, be careful to **fold** in the flour with a sharp-edged metal spoon which 'cuts' rather than with a wooden one which 'drags' the mixture.

Steam is used as a raising agent in recipes which need a large amount of liquid such as batter. It works like this. The mixture is put into a very hot oven. The liquid turns to steam. This takes up more room than the liquid and so makes the mixture rise.

Where the raising agent is steam there are two important facts to remember:

1 the recipe always contains a lot of *liquid*.
2 the mixture is always put into a *hot oven*.

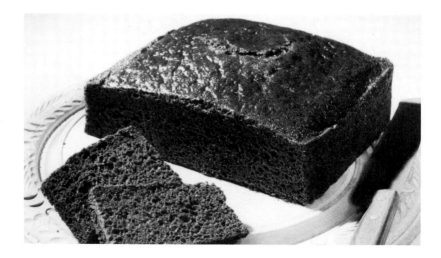

Chemical raising agents

Carbon dioxide (CO_2) is a gas. It is made when **bicarbonate of soda** is mixed with a liquid and heated. During this a chemical change takes place and sodium carbonate (washing soda) is produced. This has a bitter taste and a yellow colour.

bicarbonate   heat   sodium carbonate + carbon
of soda   →   (washing soda)   dioxide
              liquid

Adding an acid to the raising mixture changes the washing soda to another substance which is tasteless, colourless and harmless. **Cream of tartar** is a powder used to introduce an acid. Potassium hyrogen tartrate is the chemical name. It needs two parts of cream of tartar to one part of bicarbonate of soda to make the right amount of CO_2 and to change the sodium carbonate to a tasteless substance. In mixtures with a strong taste, such as gingerbread, there is no need to add cream of tartar. The taste and colour of washing soda are hidden by the strong flavour and brown colour of the mixture.

Baking powder is a useful raising agent. It is usually made from bicarbonate of soda, to produce CO_2, and one or more acid salts e.g. acid sodium pyrophosphate and acid calcium phosphate, to make it acid; a starchy powder is used as a filler.

Self-raising flour is a 'weak' flour (low in gluten strength) with a raising agent added. It was one of the first convenience foods. Enough raising agent is added for medium rich cake mixtures, such as a creaming mixture. There is too much raising agent for very rich cakes and not enough for plain mixtures such as scone dough.

Baking powder and self-raising flour do not keep for ever. They should both be kept in a dry place. Moisture will make the raising agent react and then, when it is used in a mixture, it will not produce enough CO_2 to make the mixture rise.

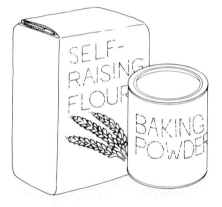

Yeast as a raising agent

Carbon dioxide is also produced when yeast is added to a mixture. Yeast is a single-celled colourless plant which multiplies by budding in the right conditions. The conditions needed are **warmth**, **food** and **moisture**. The temperature must not be too hot because yeast is killed by extreme heat.

The whole process is called **fermentation**. Enzymes both in the flour and in the yeast make this happen. During fermentation, carbon dioxide and alcohol are made in the mixture.

Yeast may be bought fresh or dried. Both are equally effective. You should mix dried yeast with a little warm liquid (from the amount given in the recipe) and leave it for about ten minutes before you add it to the mixture.

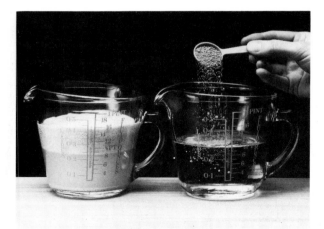

Making up dried yeast

79

Gluten

There are two proteins in flour called **gliadin** and **glutenin**. They make another protein called **gluten** when the flour is mixed with water. Gluten is stretchy and elastic. Some flours make more gluten than others. These are called **strong flours** and are best for making bread, flaky pastry and rough puff pastry. **Weak flours** are ones which make less gluten when mixed with water.

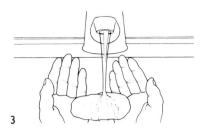

Finding out about gluten

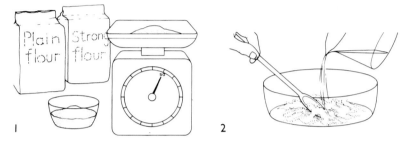

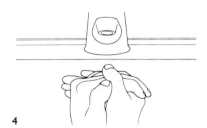

Here is an easy way to find out (a) how much gluten different flours make and (b) what the gluten is like:

1   Weigh out 50 g each of plain flour and strong flour. Keep them separate.
2   Mix each with 25-30 cm^3 water to make a stiff dough.
3   Wash each piece of dough under running water, and knead it as you do this. (This washes away the starch in the flour and leaves the gluten.)
4   Squeeze out excess water and starch.
5   Knead the dough until it is sticky.
6   Weigh each of the gluten balls and write down the weights. Is one heavier than the other? The heavier one contains more gluten. Is this the strong flour sample?
7   Stretch each piece of dough. Is one more elastic than the other? If it is, why do you think this is? Write down what you find.
8   Make sure your two pieces of dough are the same size. Bake them on a baking tray in an oven at Regulo 7 or 425°F (212°C), until they are risen and golden.
9   Are they still the same size? Is the one made from strong flour bigger than the other?

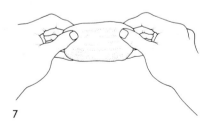

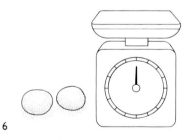

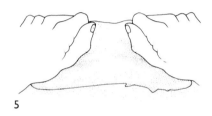

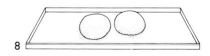

These simple experiments should show that the more gluten is made in a strong flour. This makes strong flour better for breadmaking and some pastry making where you need good elasticity and rising.

Baking

What happens to mixtures when they are prepared and baked?

Pastry

Pastries are made of flour, fats and water. Different types of pastry have different proportions of these. When flour is mixed with water, the two proteins gliadin and glutenin make gluten. Gluten makes the pastry stretchy and elastic so you can roll it.

During mixing, the fat coats the particles of flour and separates the gluten. This is what makes pastry **short**.

Air is trapped in the mixture during mixing.

What happens in the oven?

1   The starch grains in the flour swell and eventually take in so much water that they gelatinize.
2   The fat melts and is absorbed by the flour.
3   The water turns to steam. This takes up more room than the water and so the pastry rises.
4   The air expands and this makes the pastry rise more.
5   The protein coagulates and the pastry becomes crisp.
6   The pastry turns brown.

Cake mixtures

There are many different kinds of cakes. The commonest ingredients in most cakes are flour, fat, sugar and eggs.

Flour and liquid make gluten, which forms a 'network' inside the cake. This holds air, carbon dioxide (from the raising agent) and steam (from the liquid used in the recipe). The liquid added to the mixture also joins with any chemical raising agent used to produce carbon dioxide (CO_2) gas.

Fat and sugar make a cake richer and tastier. They also make the gluten network tender, which gives a light, fine texture. Creamed fat holds air.

Eggs can hold air during mixing. This helps the cake to rise.

What happens in the oven?

1   The gluten softens. CO_2 is made by the raising agent and the liquid. The air and CO_2 in the mixture expand in the hot oven. The expanding air and CO_2 make the cake rise. This stretches the gluten.
2   The proteins in the flour and egg coagulate and set the cake in the risen position.
3   The fat melts and is absorbed by the flour, giving the cakes a crumbly texture.
4   The starch in the flour swells and gelatinizes just as it does when pastry is cooked. The crust turns brown.
5   Any liquid is evaporated (turned to steam).

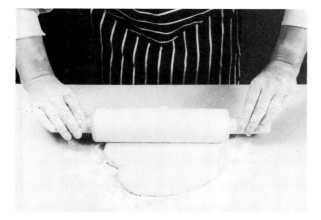

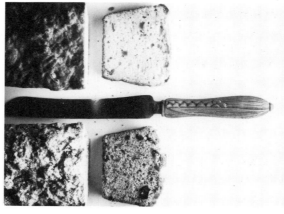

Yeast mixtures

Flour is the main ingredient used in yeast mixtures. Strong flour is best, because a lot of 'stretching' is needed to make a yeast mixture rise well.

Yeast is a raising agent. It produces carbon dioxide when it is mixed with a warm liquid and added to the other ingredients. This mixture must be left in a warm place for some time to allow the yeast to bud and produce CO_2.

Salt makes bread taste better, but too much salt slows down the action of the yeast and can spoil the mixture.

Sugar is sometimes used, but not always. A small amount can act as a 'food' for the yeast, which makes it work more quickly, though too much sugar makes it slow down. Sugar can also help the crust of the mixture to go brown.

Adding fat or oil makes the mixture shorter and helps it to keep better when cooked.

Sometimes ascorbic acid tablets are included in a yeast mixture to speed up the fermentation part of breadmaking, which can otherwise take up a long time. This is sometimes called the **Chorley Wood** method.

Steps in breadmaking

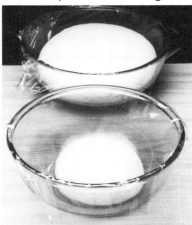

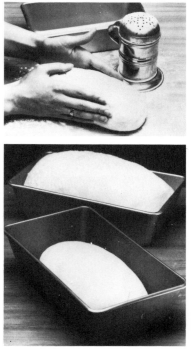

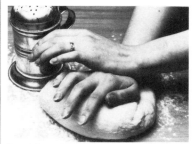

1   Flour absorbs liquid and forms gluten.

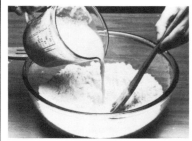

2   The dough is kneaded to develop gluten which increases its ability to stretch.

3   Fermentation (production of carbon dioxide by yeast) happens in the warm conditions.

4   The dough is 'knocked back' (re-kneaded). This spreads CO_2 throughout the mixture to give the bread an even texture.

5   The dough is shaped and proved in a warm place.

82

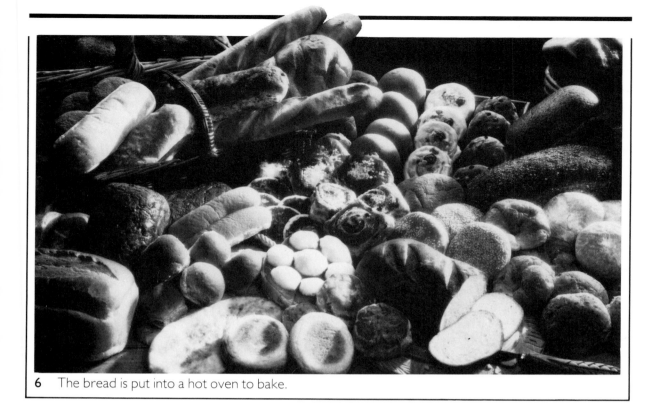

6 The bread is put into a hot oven to bake.

During baking.

a The yeast continues to make carbon dioxide at first, but then the high temperature kills it. The production of CO_2 slows down and then stops.

b The CO_2 expands with the heat.

c The gluten stretches as the gas expands and the mixture rises.

d The protein in the flour coagulates and sets the bread in the risen shape.

e The starch absorbs water, swells and gelatinizes.

f The heat drives off the alcohol produced by the yeast.

g The outside is made crisp by the heat and goes golden-brown in colour.

Things to do

1 *Study the types of 'Quick Mix' bread mixtures available. Experiment with one of them and note:*
   a *the time needed to make it up,*
   b *the texture, appearance and flavour of the bread made,*
   c *how long it stores without going stale or dry.*
   Compare your finding with someone in the class who made bread with
   a *an ordinary recipe and method*
   b *a Chorley Wood mixture and short time method.*

2 *You already know what happens to the ingredients in pastries, cakes and yeast mixtures when they are cooked. Now find a recipe for making a whisked (fatless) sponge mixture. What do you think happens in a whisked sponge mixture when it is baked?*

5.3 Food and heat

*Heat gets to food during cooking in three ways. They are: **conduction**, **convection** and **radiation**.*

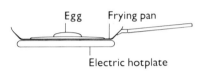

Egg   Frying pan

Electric hotplate

What is conduction?

In **conduction** heat travels direct from something hot to something cold that touches it. Some materials are better at conducting heat than others. A good conductor lets the heat pass through it easily. Most metals are good conductors and this is why pans are made of metal. Copper is a very good conductor of heat. This is why some saucepans have copper bottoms.

The handles of anything meant to hold hot liquids are made from a material that is a poor conductor of heat. Saucepans, tea pots and kettles have wooden or plastic handles. The handles do not get hot because wood and plastic are poor conductors of heat or **good insulators**.

Ovens and refrigerators have insulating material inside their walls. In the oven, this is to keep the heat in. In the refrigerator, it is to keep the heat out.

Some foods are bad conductors of heat. Meat is one, so you must allow plenty of time for the heat to get into the middle of a thick piece of meat when it is cooking. Bone is a better conductor of heat. This means that sometimes meat in a joint may cook more quickly near the bone.

Water and steam are better conductors of heat than air. This makes moist methods of cooking, such as boiling and stewing, quicker than baking.

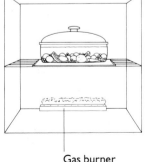

Gas oven

Gas burner

What is convection?

In **convection**, heat travels because of the movement of molecules when they are heated. Hot air and hot liquid rise, and cold air or liquid move in to take their place at the bottom. A good example is water being heated in a saucepan. The hot water next to the hotplate at the bottom of the saucepan rises to the top. It cools because the air touches it. Then the cooled water drops to the bottom again. This is a continuous movement. It is called a **convection current**.

Ovens are heated by convection currents of air. The hot air rises from the heating elements. It cools down at the top of the oven and then drops again. In the same way, refrigerators have convection currents of warm air rising to the freezer unit. The air is cooled there and then the cold air drops.

Boiling, steaming and deep fat frying all use convection currents to bring heat to food. Water, fat and steam also **conduct** heat better than air, and this can speed up cooking.

What is radiation?

Radiation is a way of carrying heat in rays or waves, which heat anything in their path. Heat is radiated from a grill (**radiant heat**) onto food in the grill pan, and as the food absorbs the heat it is cooked. There is shiny reflective plate behind the source of heat to direct all the radiant heat onto the food.

Radiant heat is important in oven cooking as well as in grilling and toasting.

Radiant heat also helps to keep food hot in a **vacuum flask** (or thermos flask). The container is made of two layers of glass. The inner layer is shiny. This silvery wall reflects the rays of heat back into the food and keeps it hot. There is no air (a vacuum) between the two layers so heat is not lost by conduction or convection either.

If cold food is put into the flask, the food stays cold even on a hot day.

A plastic top (a poor conductor of heat) stops heat getting in or out through the opening of the flask.

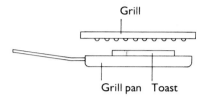

Grill

Grill pan Toast

How air, water and oil pass on heat

Air transmits (passes on) heat to food mainly by convection and radiation. This happens in roasting, grilling and baking.

Water transmits heat to food mainly by convection and conduction. This happens in boiling, stewing, simmering, poaching, braising and steaming.

Oil transmits heat to food by convection and conduction as in frying and sautéing.

Things to do

1 *How is heat passed on in the following?*
   a *toasting bread*
   b *boiling vegetables,*
   c *pressure cooking a stew.*

2 *With your teacher's help, find out which are the coldest and the warmest parts of the refrigerator.*

3 *Describe four different methods of cooking meat. Say how the heat is carried to the meat from the heat source.*

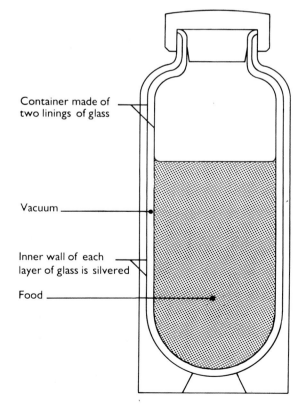

Container made of two linings of glass

Vacuum

Inner wall of each layer of glass is silvered

Food

5.4 Cookers and ovens

Cookers and food

Food is cooked on the **hob**, under the **grill** or in the **oven** of a cooker. This is how the different parts of the cooker cook the food:

1   Hob — the heat underneath gets to the pan by convection (through the air) and conduction (through the metal base of the pan). The pan must be in full contact with the hob. On electric cookers, the pan should be the same size as the hob. On gas cookers, the flames must not go up the side of the pan.

2   Grill — the grill gets red-hot and gives out radiant heat which is reflected on to the food by a back cover or highly polished reflector.

3   Oven — heat circulates in the oven by convection currents. Heat also passes along the oven shelves to the food by conduction. Some heat also radiates from the sides of the oven, particularly in electric ovens.

Microwave cooking

In conduction, convection and radiation, heat gets into food gradually from the outside. **Microwave** cooking is different. Microwaves are a special sort of radiation that makes the molecules of liquid in the food vibrate (move about) very fast. This movement produces **heat**, which cooks the food. The whole of the food, not just the outside, heats up very quickly.

Microwaves can penetrate food only to a depth of 4-5 cm. This means that small pieces of food are cooked through very quickly. Larger pieces take longer, because where the microwaves cannot penetrate, the heat is *conducted* through the food.

How microwave cookers work

The microwave energy is generated by a **magnetron**. The energy is taken into the cooker by a metal lined tube. The waves enter from the top and a wave stirrer moves very slowly to send the waves to each part of the cooker. It is the stirrer which ensures that the food cooks evenly. The door and the seal of the cooker are specially made to stop any microwaves getting out.

Glass, china and paper let microwaves go through them to the food without getting hot themselves (except by conduction from the hot food). Metals do *not* let the waves go through them to the food; they reflect the microwaves back against the cooker walls, causing damage to the cooker and leaving the food uncooked. So you cannot use metal cooking pots.

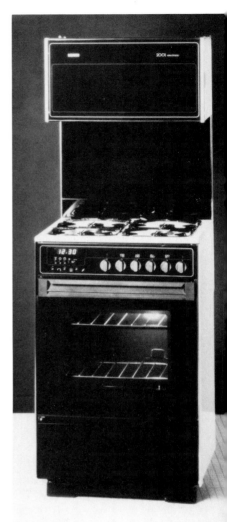

A gas cooker

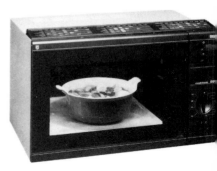

A microwave oven

Microwave ovens save time and fuel. Food does not go brown or crisp in a microwave oven, but this can be done by a special browning dish. Some microwave ovens have a turntable to make sure the food is cooked evenly.

Fan assisted ovens

In fan assisted ovens the convection currents of hot air are forced around the oven by a fan. The oven may be heated by gas or electricity in the usual way.

The oven cooks food more quickly and gets slightly hotter, so this helps to save fuel. Manufacturers usually recommend a lower setting (about 25°C less) than for an oven without a fan, and a shorter cooking time.

The movement of air may equalize the temperature inside the oven so that it is not **zoned** (slightly hotter in some places than others). This has not been finally proved. However, it is easier to get even results from a 'bulk bake' in a fan assisted oven, probably because the temperature is constant at any shelf position.

Hot air ovens

These ovens have a round electrical element with a fan in the middle. The element heats up and the fan blows the hot air around the oven. In front of the fan is a plate with vents in it. The hot air is blown through the vents. This means that the temperature is the same on each shelf.

Cramic glass hobs

The heat sources for these hobs are normal radiant elements in a fireclay bowl. These hobs work at a lower temperature than conventional 'red ring' elements. This can make it difficult to 'seal' food and get a crisp brown surface on meat. Some people think that ceramic hobs use less electricity than other hobs.

The new magnetic induction hobs use ceramic glass in a different way. There are no heating elements in these hobs. The ceramic surface does not get hot. The pan is the heating agent. This is what happens. An electric generator underneath the hob produces a magnetic field just above the hob surface. When a metal pan is put into this magnetic field the power makes both the pan and the food in it heat up very quickly. This is quicker than any of the sorts of direct heat we have looked at.

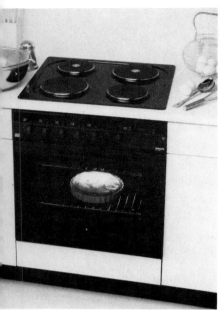

An electric cooker with a fan assisted oven

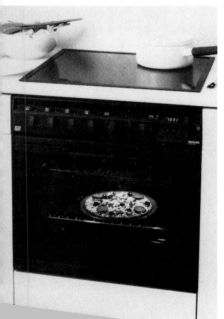

An electric cooker with a ceramic hob

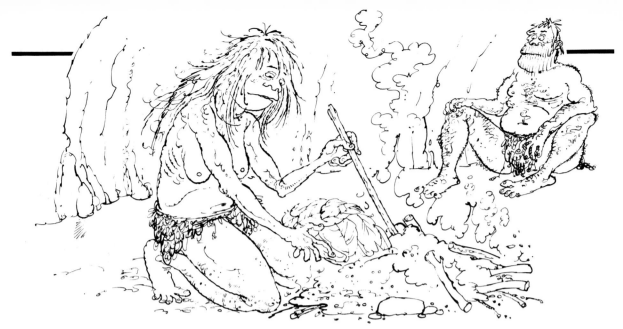

Slow cooking

'Slow cooking' is getting more popular because people need to save fuel, and in many homes everyone is out during the day. The idea of slow cooking is not a new one. In the Stone Age people wrapped pieces of meat in large leaves and left them in hot ashes to cook overnight. Old fashioned solid fuel kitchen ranges always had a slow oven. So have the 'Aga' ranges of today.

The 'hay-box' method of cooking used during World War II is a sort of slow cooking. A casserole or stew is brought to the boil on a cooker and then put into a box full of hay. The hay acts as an insulator and prevents heat loss and the food cooks slowly all day.

How slow cooking works

It is important to give food enough time when you slow cook it, to make sure it is cooked through properly. Food that can be cooked like this is held at a pre-set, constant temperature (between 71°C and 82°C) for a long time.

Less liquid is used in slow cooking recipes. The mixture doesn't boil, and moisture doesn't evaporate. All the juices and flavour of the food are kept in – the food cooks in its own moisture.

People say that the food shrinks less in slow cooking. The slow heat and moisture gradually break down the fatty tissue in tougher meat and make it more tender. So the cook can use cheaper cuts of meat.

Advantages of slow cooking	Disadvantages of slow cooking
1 Saves fuel.	1 Food has to be prepared in the morning and not everyone likes the smell of, e.g. onions and meat browning for a stew while they are eating breakfast.
2 Food can be left for a long time.	
3 The working cook can come home to a hot meal.	
4 A meal can be prepared for an invalid or old person to have later in the day.	2 Some vegetables, e.g. red kidney beans, may not cook completely at the temperature in the slow cooker. This may mean that the toxin (the poisonous substance inside them) is not destroyed.
5 Slow cooking pots don't take up much room. They are useful in a tiny flat or 'bedsit'.	
6 The food does not dry, and meat is tenderized.	

Slow cooking pots

You can buy many different types of slow cooking pot in the shops. They are usually made of stoneware, which is a poor conductor of heat. The stoneware is well insulated and has an electric heating element in the base.

The heat travels to the food by conduction through the pot from the element. Because the stoneware pot is a poor conductor of heat the transfer of heat is slow. This keeps the food at a constant temperature and lets it cook slowly. The food can be left in the pot for a long time.

The pots work on a small amount of electricity. They are called **low wattage** appliances. In fact, the manufacturers say that they burn no more electricity than a 60 watt electric light bulb. This obviously saves fuel.

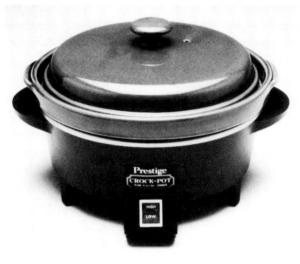

A slow cooking pot

Slow cooking ovens

Gas ovens can be made with a special slow cooking setting. The manufacturers have developed a special thermostat valve. When the 'S' setting is used, the oven only burns enough gas to heat it to between 80°C and 110°C. The oven works normally when the 'S' setting is not used.

During slow cooking, the heat in the oven is zoned. The temperature differences are small; the lowest temperature at the bottom is 75°C, and the highest at the top is 110°C. The manufacturers say that even the lowest temperature is hot enough to kill any bacteria. They also say that the slow cooking setting can be used to cook several dishes at the same time.

Things to do

1   *How useful would a microwave oven be to someone who owns a freezer? Make a chart to show how it could be used.*

2   *Find out how microwave ovens are used in cafés and canteens. Why do you think they are useful?*

3   *There are some disadvantages to slow cooking. What are they?*

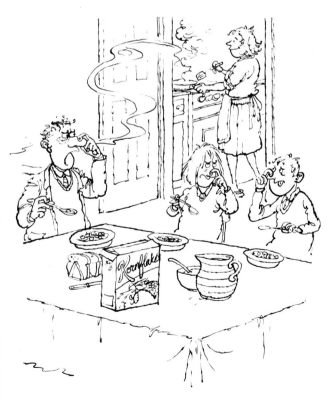

5.5 Cooking materials

Today casserole dishes and pans are available in so many different materials that it is difficult to choose which one to buy. It helps if you know the advantages and disadvantages of the different materials used.

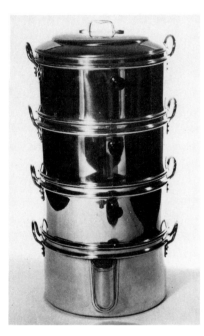

Aluminium

Aluminium is a good conductor of heat. This means that fuel is used economically and the food is cooked evenly. Aluminium is a light metal, so it is easy to lift. Aluminium pans can be made with a thick base which helps to spread the heat evenly; this is important when the pan is used on an electric hob. Pans with a thick base are called **ground base** saucepans.

Aluminium stains very easily, but it can be cleaned with steel wool pads. The pads are soaked with a pink material called **jewellers' rouge**. This is what makes the metal shine after cleaning.

Stainless steel

Stainless steel is made from a mixture of iron, nickel (so that it does not corrode) and chromium (for extra strength).

Stainless steel is a poor conductor of heat, so stainless steel pans usually have a disc of copper or aluminium in the base.

Pans made from stainless steel last a long time and stay bright, but they are usually expensive.

Pyroceram

Pyroceram is a ceramic material (a kind of pottery) developed to stand the tremendous temperature changes in space rockets! Dishes made of this can be taken straight from the freezer and heated straight away without cracking. Handles can be taken off for storage.

These dishes may be used on top of the cooker or in the oven, and are very attractive oven-to-table ware. They hold the heat longer than metal pans, so the food will continue to cook after they have been taken from the heat.

Vitreous enamelled steel

Steel cannot be used for making pans without a coating, because it

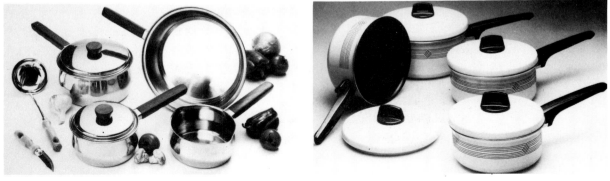

rusts. The coating used for covering a steel saucepan inside and outside is **vitreous enamel**. This material is made from glass ground up into tiny particles, which are fused (melted) on to the metal. Iron and aluminium can be treated in this way too. The enamel makes a hard, hygienic surface that does not scratch easily. It can be finished in different colours and designs.

Enamelled steel has some disadvantages. Steel is an uneven conductor of heat, which may cause 'hot spots' and sticking. The enamel chips easily.

The British Vitreous Enamel Development Council has drawn up quality guidelines for steel and cast iron cookware coated with vitreous enamel. Pans made to meet this standard may be labelled **Vitramel**.

Cast iron

There are many attractive cooking pots made of cast iron.

Iron is a good conductor and retainer of heat. This makes it very good for long, slow cooking and means that less fuel is needed when cast iron cooking pots are used.

Iron rusts easily. To stop this, the pans and pots should be coated with vitreous enamel.

The main disadvantage of cast iron pans and casseroles is that they are very heavy.

Non-stick coatings

Pans with non-stick linings are very popular because they are so easy to clean.

The non-stick finish is usually made from polytetrafluorethylene, or p.t.f.e for short. The coating is non-porous (that means that food cannot seep through it). This is what makes food come out of the pan so easily.

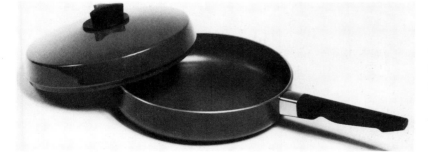

There are many different kinds of non-stick coating. The more recent ones last longer than the early ones, if they are properly used. Follow the cleaning instructions carefully.

Ceramic ware

There are many different kinds of ceramic cooking pots.

Stoneware is made from natural clay which is 'fired' at very high temperatures. It is a very strong and can stand high temperatures, but it is not 'flame-proof' (you can't use it on top of the cooker). The famous Denbyware dishes are made from this.

Earthenware pots are made of earth or red clay. They are porous, and absorb fat and smells from cooking. Many earthenware casseroles come from the continent, and the glaze on some of these has more lead and cadmium in it than is allowed in this country. There has been some disagreement whether these pots are safe to use. Some British firms now make earthenware dishes to the British Standard, which says how much lead and cadmium there can be in the glaze.

Glass ceramics are made of glass which can stand high temperatures. An example of this is the glass we call **pyrex**. This is **borosilicate** glass made from 80% silver sand, with small amounts of alumina, borax, boractic acid and salt. This mixture gives Pyrex its good heat resistance.

Pyrex is only a moderately good conductor of heat. Have you noticed that if you line a Pyrex plate or dish with pastry, that after cooking there is a ring of slightly undercooked pastry in the centre? This happens because the Pyrex does not conduct the heat right to the centre of the dish.

The heat is conducted better if the dish is put on a baking tray, because a metal baking tray is a good conductor of heat. However, Pyrex containers probably transfer radiant heat better than metal ones. This means you need to watch food cooked in a Pyrex dish to stop it from getting too brown on the outside.

Things to do

1 *What materials are the pans and casseroles in the home economics room made from? Are the handles and bases of the pans made from the same material? If not, why do you think this is?*

2 *What is the advantage of a non-stick pan in 'low-fat' cooking? Carry out a simple experiment by frying an egg:*
   a in a frying pan without a non-stick lining,
   b in a non-stick frying pan.
   Do you need the same amount of fat in each?

3 *Try to find some casseroles made from pyroceram. What instructions are given about their use and care? Do you think they are useful? If so, why?*

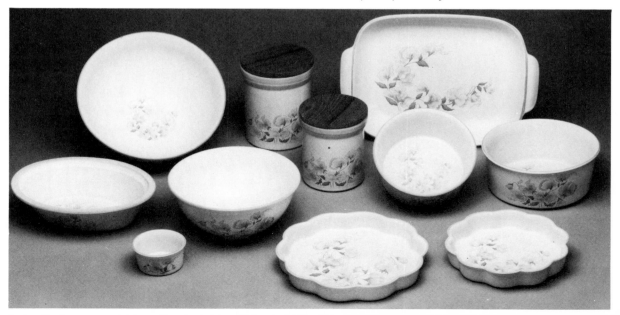

Recap 5

Pair up the 'heads' and 'tails' of the following sentences correctly:

1 Food...transmits heat to food by convection and conduction.
2 Yeast...is made when flour is mixed with water.
3 Gluten...is made from flour, fat and water.
4 Pastry...is a biological raising agent.
5 Oil...keeps better after cooking.

Answer the following questions with one or more sentences:

6 How can we stop vitamin C from being destroyed?
7 What is convection?
8 How does a vacuum flask work?
9 Why is microwave cooking different from other methods of cooking?
10 How does slow cooking work?

11 Compare how long it takes to cook each of the following in (a) an ordinary oven and (b) in a microwave oven:
   a baked potato in jacket,
   b two baked potatoes in jackets,
   c chicken casserole,
   d gingerbread.

12 Write a summary of how the different raising agents used in baking work. Unit 5.2 will help you. Include these words:
   Gas...physical...expand...volume...heat...liquid...oven...fold.
   Cut out pictures from magazines and do drawings to illustrate your work.

13 Plan a selection of dishes which you think could be cooked in an oven with an 'S' setting. Say where each dish should be put in the oven.

14 Find out from the label on a new piece of 'non-stick' linings. Draw up a chart to show what you must and must not do when cleaning these materials. Call your chart 'How to care for non-stick pans'.

15 Compare the sizes and prices of a set of saucepans made from:
   a aluminium,
   b stainless steel,
   c stainless steel with copper base,
   d cast iron (enamelled),
   e enamelled steel.
   Which set would you choose as best value for money if you were setting up home? Give reasons.

16 Describe the effects of
   a moist methods of cooking and
   b dry methods of cooking
   on the nutrients in specific foods.

17 Assess the use and value of dishes made from:
   a pyrex,
   b pyroceram.

6 Food, hygiene and storage

6.1 Food and bacteria

*In the air all around us are minute organisms called **bacteria**. We sometimes refer to them as germs. They are so small that we can only see them with a microscope. Some of them are harmful and can cause **food poisoning**. So we need to take great care to ensure that the food we prepare is safe or **uncontaminated**.*

What bacteria do

Bacteria need **warmth**, **food** and **moisture** to live. When all these conditions happen at once, the bacteria will multiply. Bacteria in food can be harmful in two ways:

1 Bacteria can be in food when it is eaten. They die in the body and then release a poison which irritates the stomach and the bowels. This causes sickness, diarrhoea and stomach pains. This is called **infective** food poisoning. One type of bacteria that causes this is salmonella.

2 Bacteria can grow on certain foods such as meat, cream, milk and custard. They produce **poisons** and these cause sickness and diarrhoea when the food is eaten. This is called **toxic** food poisoning. The bacteria that make poisons are Staphylococci, *Clostridium welchii* and *Clostridium botulinus*. *Clostridium botulinus* causes **botulism**, a very serious illness which can kill you. This type of food poisoning is rare.

The table shows the foods most likely to be infected ('at risk'), and the symptoms the infections cause in you.

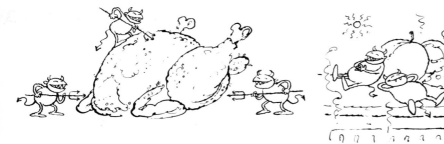
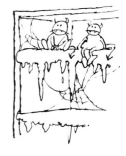

Bacteria responsible	Foods 'at risk'	Symptoms
Salmonella	Sliced cooked meat, meat pies, duck eggs, cream, shellfish	Sickness and diarrhoea. Lasts 1-7 days. Unpleasant, but not usually serious.
Clostridium welchii	Gravy, pre-cooked meat, stews	Severe stomach pains. Lasts 1-2 days.
Staphylococci	Meat pies, sliced meats, gravy, ice-cream	Severe sickness. Unpleasant, but not normally serious.
Clostridium botulinus	Incorrectly handled and processed canned meat, vegetables and fish.	Double vision. Difficulty in swallowing and breathing. Often fatal. If not, recovery is slow.

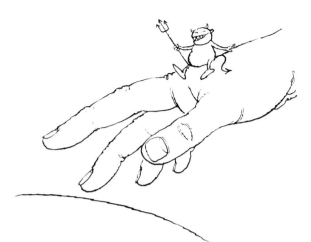

How do bacteria get to food?

Some of the causes of food contamination are:

1 **People** — personal hygiene is very important. Bacteria are present both inside and outside our bodies and harmful ones can be transferred to food by careless people.
2 **Vermin** and **flies** — rats and mice can carry salmonella bacteria on their bodies. So can flies.
3 **Food** itself — bacteria may be there already. E.g. salmonella bacteria can be in meat from all animals, in duck eggs and in milk powders.

How to make sure cooked food is safe to eat

Perishable food should be cooked as **fresh** as possible, and **thoroughly** because heat kills bacteria.

Certain foods need extra careful treatment. These include sausages, meat pies and similar 'prepared' foods. These are **manufactured** foods. If the conditions during manufacture are not as hygienic as they should be, the products may become contaminated. To ensure that any bacteria present are destroyed, the foods must be cooked at a temperature high enough to kill bacteria.

Remember that *warmth* and *moisture* encourage bacteria to grow. Because of this it is very important to cool cooked food as quickly as possible if it is not going to be eaten straight away. The food should also be covered while it is cooling. When cool, the food should be put into the fridge as soon as possible.

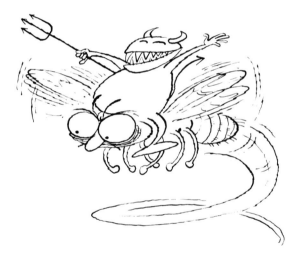

Reheating food

Any reheated food or dish must be **thoroughly heated**. It should be heated to a **high temperature** and **right through to the middle**. This is because bacteria can grow in food during storage.

Gravy, sauces, soups and stocks are ideal food for bacteria to grow in. Extra care should be taken when reheating any of these. None of them should be stored for future use unless they are carefully deep frozen. Stock may be kept for a number of days provided it is boiled up everyday.

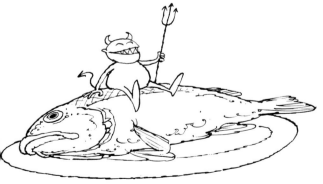

Things to do

1 *Finding out about bacteria*

Do **not** carry out this activity in the home economics room because you may contaminate the kitchen surfaces. Instead do your test in the biology laboratory.

Make up a jelly using a stock cube and some gelatin. Use about 30 g gelatin in ½ litre of water for a good 'set'. Clean six petri dishes and pour some of the liquid into each. Cover them immediately and leave them to set.

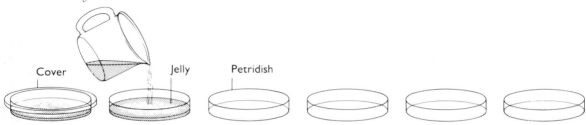

Now number the dishes 1 — 6 and treat them as follows:

1 Leave covered as a 'control' to compare with the other dishes.
2 Press washed fingers on to the jelly.
3 Press unwashed fingers on to the jelly.
4 Put three or four human hairs on the jelly.
5 Cough on to the jelly surface.
6 Press an unwashed tea towel or dish cloth on to the jelly surface.

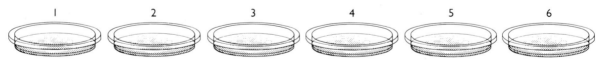

Cover all the dishes and leave them in a warm place for four days. The temperature should be between 30°C and 40°C.

After four days look at the dishes. Write down what has happened in each dish. What do your results tell you about bacteria, and the importance of hygiene?

Caution: When you have finished with the dishes, ask your biology teacher to destroy the jelly. The jelly will probably be burnt in a special incinerator for safety.

2 What should you do with left-over trifle? Why do you think that extra care should be taken with this kind of dish?

3 Design a poster to show people the dangers of contaminated food. Call your poster 'Warning! Bacteria at work'. Make it as visual as you can.

6.2 Food and spoilage

*Fruit and vegetables that are not picked after they have ripened go on ripening until they are rotten. Enzymes cause the ripening. We say this kind of food spoilage is caused by **enzyme action**. The main causes of food spoilage however, are tiny creatures called **micro-organisms**. These may be yeasts, moulds or bacteria.*

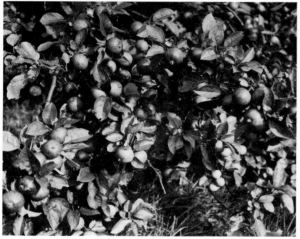

Once it is ripe fruit will continue to ripen until it is rotten

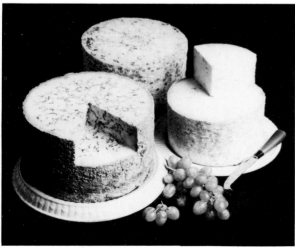

Moulds grow on the surface of foods such as cheese

What do micro-organisms do?

Not all micro-organisms are harmful. For example, some cheeses and yoghurt get their flavour from micro-organism rowth.

Micro-organisms need three conditions to live and thrive. These are: **warmth**, **food** and **moisture**.

Micro-organisms cannot grow when any of these three things are missing. This is an important principle used in **preserving** food. When you freeze or dry food you are using this principle.

The organisms are tiny — this is what 'micro' means. They can only be seen under a microscope.

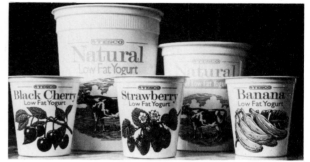

Yoghurt gets its flavour from micro-organisms

What kills micro-organisms?

Bacteria are the most difficult micro-organisms to destroy. They are killed by **heat** and made inactive by **cold**. Bacteria multiply very rapidly in warm, moist conditions. Some are more resistant to heat than others. In acidic food such as fruit, bacteria can be killed at the temperature of boiling water. In non-acidic food such as meat and vegetables, the bacteria can still be active at temperatures above that of boiling water.

Moulds usually grow on the surface of foods such as cheese, bread, fruit and jelly. Moulds are destroyed by **heat**.

Yeasts are always present in air. They are similar to moulds but grow on sugary foods. You can see bubbles of carbon dioxide (CO_2) on the food as the yeast changes the sugar in the food to carbon dioxide and alcohol. This is called **fermentation**. Yeasts can be killed by temperatures slightly below that of boiling water.

Preventing spoilage

To keep food fresh for any length of time you must not let micro-organisms grow. We know that micro-organisms need warmth, food and moisture to grow. We also know that they are destroyed by heat. The way we stop micro-organisms from growing is by **preserving** food.

There are several different ways of doing this. the table below shows how each method works.

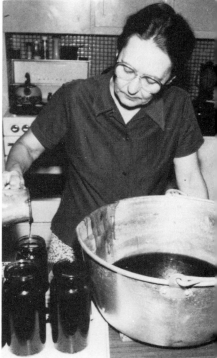

Making jam

Method	How does it work?
Canning and bottling	Extreme heat is applied to the food to kill existing micro-organisms. The container is made airtight (a vacuum is produced) so that no more bacteria can enter or live in the food.
Drying	Moisture is removed. Food is put in the sun or in a current of warm air until all the moisture has gone. The food will keep for a long time if it is kept dry, but as soon as liquid is added to it, it becomes perishable.
Freezing	Warmth is removed. However, remember that freezing or cold conditions do not kill micro-organisms — the cold **inactivates** them and stops them growing. When the food is thawed, the micro-organisms grow more rapidly to make up for lost time.
Accelerated freeze-drying (AFD)	Food is frozen and then dried. The ice on the food can be changed into water vapour without first melting to liquid (called **sublimation**) in this method. It is rather expensive but has many advantages. It is used for 'Surprise' peas, some instant coffee granules, some packaged curries and chow mein. Large pieces of food such as steaks can be freeze-dried whole. Delicate foods such as prawns can be freeze-dried without spoiling their appearance and texture.

Using preservatives

There are other ways of stopping food from spoiling. You can use substances called **preservatives**. Micro-organisms can't live and multiply in these substances, so the food is safe to keep.

Smoking is one of the oldest methods of preserving. Food such as fish is hung in the smoke from burning wood. This kills the micro-orgasnisms and prevents further contamination.

Sugar solution is another preservative. It is used when making jams and jellies. Careful measuring of ingredients is important in jam and jelly making. 60% of the total weight must be sugar for the jam or jelly to keep.

Vinegar and **spices** are also preservatives. Their use in this way is called **pickling**. The solution must be concentrated (strong) enough. Choose a reliable recipe and method, and measure the ingredients carefully when preparing pickles.

Permitted preservatives are added to some foods during manufacture. **Sulphur dioxide** (SO_2) is used for preserving fruit and fruit juices, jams and sausages. The word 'permitted' is used because, by law, only certain chemicals may be added to food. Those that are allowed are called 'permitted'.

Why do we preserve food?

Food is preserved to:

1. prevent waste,
2. use up a glut e.g. from a big crop of apples or plums,
3. add variety to the diet, because preserved food can be saved to eat out of season,
4. make transport easier — packages and cans are easier to carry than fresh food,
5. store for emergency use e.g. when someone is ill and can't shop, or when unexpected visitors call.

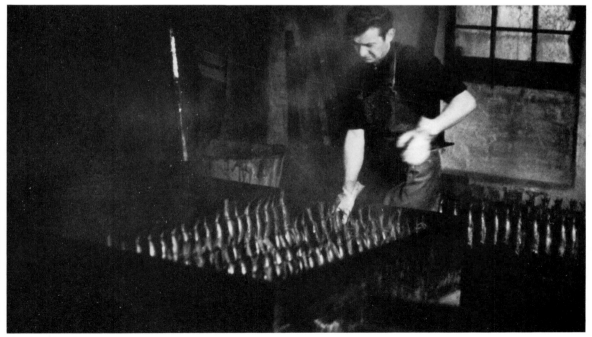

Smoking herrings

A summary of methods of preserving food

Method used	Fact on which the method is based	Products
Drying	Micro-organisms cannot grow without water.	Dried vegetables and fruits, milk, freeze-dried whole meals, coffee granules, vegetables
Canning and bottling	Heat kills organisms. Containers are sealed so micro-organisms cannot get in.	Canned meat, canned and bottled fruit and vegetables
Freezing	Micro-organisms cannot grow and multiply in cold conditions.	Quick-frozen vegetables, fish, meat, cooked dishes. Other frozen food e.g. ice-cream
Chemicals and other preservatives	Preservative kills micro-organisms and prevents further contamination.	Vinegar: pickles, chutney Sugar: jams and jellies Sulphur dioxide: fruit juices, jams,

Things to do

1 *Find examples of foods preserved by accelerated freeze-drying (AFD) at the supermarket. What are the advantages of this method of preserving food?*

2 *Compare the length of time freeze-dried food takes to cook with the time it takes to cook the same dish using fresh ingredients.*

3 *How much of the food we eat is preserved? Make a list based on what you had to eat yesterday.*

6.3 Nutrition and preserved food

Dried food

Vitamin C is destroyed by most drying methods. Accelerated freeze-drying conserves some of the vitamin. Some riboflavin and thiamin is also lost. Dried milk and dried eggs are only slightly less nutritious than the fresh products.

Dried foods must be packed carefully to stop them getting damp. Sometimes packets of **silica gel** or other **drying agents** are included in packets of dried food.

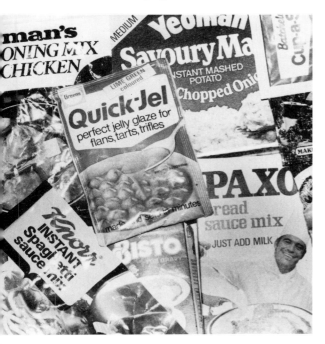

Canned food

Some vitamins are lost in canning. Often the loss is no more than in home cooking however, and it can be less.

The food used for canning is very fresh and in top n¼ dition. So very few nutrients have been lost by poor storage or by using food 'past its best'.

The amount of vitamin C (ascorbic acid) in food is reduced by canning and reduced further by storage. However, if the can is stored in a cool place, t¼ amin C destruction is slower.

More thiamin is lost from meat during canning than would be lost if the meat was cooked normally.

There are two points you should remember:

1 Apart from the loss of vitamin C and thiamin, canned foods are just as good nutritionally as fresh foods.
2 Canned foods may contain more nutrients than some fresh foods. This is because fruit and vegetables are usually canned very soon after picking. Fresh food which is not in top condition or has been stored badly is bound to lose a lot of nutrients.

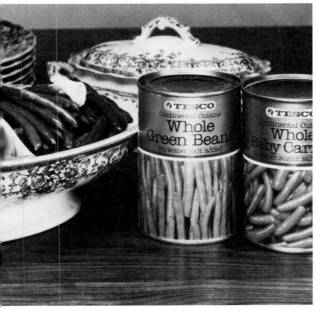

High temperature, short time canning

By increasing the temperatures used in canning the time taken can be reduced. This process is called **high temperature, short time canning** or **HTST**. It is also called **aseptic canning**.

Less thiamin is lost in this method than in normal canning but at the moment only liquid or puréed food can be treated in this way.

Frozen food

The nutritive value of frozen food compares well with fresh food. It is better than any other processed food, particularly if the food has been 'fast frozen'. The nutritive value of accelerated freeze-dried food also compares well with fresh food.

Frozen fruit and vegetables may have more nutrients than fresh fruit and vegetables. This is because the fruit and vegetables are usually frozen soon after picking.

Fruit keeps its vitamin C very well when it is frozen but some may be lost when it is stored. This is particularly likely if the temperature rises above −17.8°C. Because of this it is important to check the temperature of your freezer regularly. Make sure you buy your ready-frozen food from a shop where staff check the temperature of the frozen food cabinets.

Food such as strawberries or whole fish can be frozen very quickly in liquid nitrogen. This is a fairly new process which may preserve more of the nutrients because the freezing is almost instantaneous. This method will probably be used for other highly perishable foods eventually. It is called **cryogenic freezing**. This process helps the food to keep its original shape and appearance.

Things to do

1 *Find out how much one portion of peas would cost if bought in each of the following forms:*

   a *tinned,*
   b *dried,*
   c *accelerated freeze-dried,*
   d *frozen,*
   e *fresh.*
   Compare the different forms. Mention the following:
   Preparation time…appearance when cooked …texture, colour and flavour…ease of storage.

2 *Have you ever found packets of silica gel or other drying agents in packets of dried food? What foods were they in?*

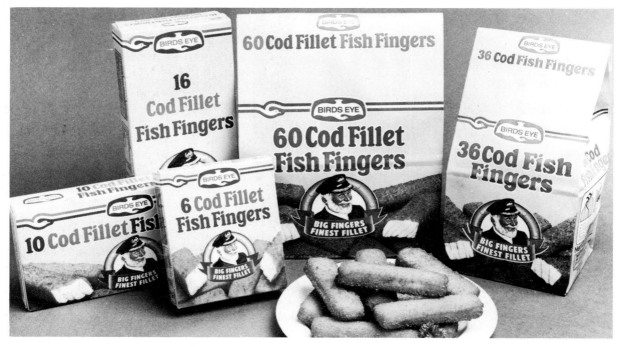

6.4 Kitchen hygiene

Personal hygiene is very important when dealing with food. Kitchen hygiene is equally important.

Keeping the kitchen clean

Floors, walls and working surfaces should be made of a material which can be cleaned easily. They should be washed frequently with hot, soapy water.

Wash working surfaces thoroughly after food has been prepared on them. Check that your working surface is clean before you start preparing food. Keep all equipment spotlessly clean. Pay special attention to the parts which are difficult to reach such as inside the bottoms of saucepans and between the prongs of forks. If you have pets, their food and food bowls must be stored and cleaned separately from the family's food and china.
Remember: pets carry bacteria both on and in their bodies.

To have a hygienic kitchen it is also important to:

1 store food safely, and
2 dispose of waste efficiently and safely.

Food storage

Because bacteria need warmth and moisture to grow, food should be stored in **cool** and **dry** conditions.

A well ventilated, clean and cool **larder** is an ideal place for many foods. A **refrigerator** is necessary for storing the most perishable foods, such as meat, fish, cheese, eggs, milk and some fruits and vegetables. It is particularly useful in summer.

Bacteria do not grow and multiply in the cold. Note that they are not killed by the cold, they are just **'inactivated'** or slowed down. So the rate at which they spoil food is also slowed down.

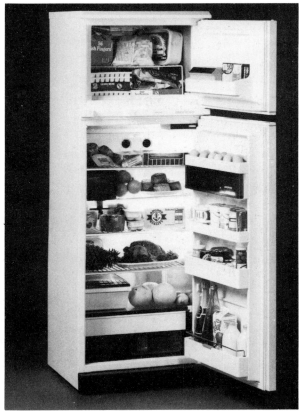

...and in a refrigerator

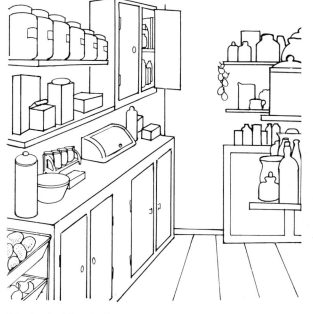

Storing food in a larder...

Refrigeration

The refrigerator has 'zones' of cold. The centre of the refrigerator is usually about 4°C. Under the ice box or freezer compartment the temperature is about 1-2°C. Door storage temperature is usually between 5°C and 8°C. The freezer compartment is the coldest part. The temperature is usually between -6°C and -15°C. The table gives you some more useful facts about refrigeration.

Fact	Using the fact
1 In the freezer compartment **evaporation** takes place and this causes cooling. 2 Cold air is heavier than warm air. Cold air falls to the bottom and warm air rises.	The coldest zone is just under the ice-box. Food that perishes easily should be stored here e.g. meat, bacon, sausages.
3 The moving air absorbs moisture.	Uncovered food will dry. Salads lose their crispness if not covered. This is why most fridges have a 'crisper' drawer.
4 Air needs to circulate freely for a fridge to work efficiently.	The fridge should not be packed too full.
5 Warm air entering the fridge will raise the temperature.	Open the door as little as possible and for as short a time as possible. Hot food must be cooled before putting it in the fridge.

Star ratings

The freezer compartments of modern refrigerators are marked with **stars**. Most packets of freezer food are also marked with one, two or three stars, showing how long they may be stored frozen. You match up the number of stars on your freezer compartment with the number on the food packet and then you know how long you can keep the food.

Here is the star-rating system:

Things to do

1 *Investigate the frozen foods in your local supermarket. Compare the star ratings of different foods.*

2 *Which of the following materials would be easiest to clean as a working surface? Wood...ceramic...stainless steel...formica. Give reasons.*

*	(one star)	maximum temperature -6°C	Frozen food can be stored for 1 week.
**	(two stars)	maximum temperature -12°C	Frozen food can be stored for 1 month.
***	(three stars)	maximum temperature -15°C	Frozen food can be stored for 3 months.

6.5 Waste disposal

An average home in the UK produces about 50 kg of household refuse every week. The diagram below shows you what sort of things we dispose of.

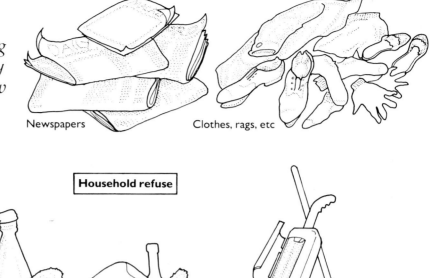

Newspapers

Clothes, rags, etc

Household refuse

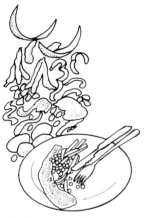

Food waste: peelings, food left on plates, stale food

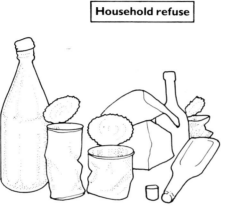

Food packages: paper, cardboard, plastic, tins and jars

Dust from vacuum cleaner and sweeper
Ash from fires

Kitchen waste

Kitchen waste is the waste or refuse frm storing, preparing and cooking food. It includes peelings from fruit and vegetables, food left on plates, stale food and packaging from food such as cardboard, tins and jars.

This is how you should deal with waste in the kitchen:

1 Use a pedal bin. Empty it regularly and wash it out thoroughly with disinfectant each time. Plastic bin liners are very useful. Seal them tightly before putting them in the dustbin.
2 Keep the waste dry.
3 Always wrap vegetable peelings in newspaper before putting them in the bin. Use them for compost instead of throwing them away if you can.

4 Use a dustbin with a tight-fitting lid.
5 Wash out the dustbin regularly with detergent. Keep it out of the sun.
6 Stand your dustbin on bricks to let the air circulate underneath it.

It is a good idea to try to avoid too much waste. You can do this by:

1 Choosing perishable food carefully. Buy fruit and vegetables that are unbruised and undamaged. Store food in a cool place. This will stop you having to throw out food because it has gone bad.
2 Re-using as much waste paper as you can.
3 Using food cartons for other things once they are empty.

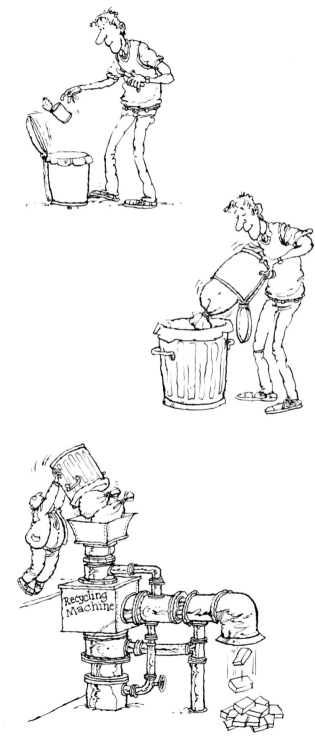

Getting rid of the waste

Kitchen waste is usually collected in a pedal bin. This is then emptied into a dustbin which is cleared every week. In country areas the refuse collection may be less frequent. It may be worth burning waste paper and cardboard. Vegetable matter can be used as compost.

Local authorities treat the disposal of our waste in different ways. For example, one authority is changing the refuse into fuel. This is called **recycling** and means that the waste is not wasted at all! This is a very good idea. In some places voluntary groups like the Scouts or Friends of the Earth will collect and recycle waste paper.

Disposing of waste without dustbins

Some kitchen sinks have **waste disposal units** connected to them. They will dispose of everything except bottles, cans and some plastics. The unit is a 'grinder' which grinds the waste so that it can be flushed down the drain with water.

In some flats there is an arrangement called a **chute**. The waste from each flat is put down the chute and it is collected from a central point at the bottom.

In some areas the local council supplies **heavy duty sacks** that fit onto a metal frame. You do not need a dustbin then. The refuse collectors just take away the sacks.

Things to do

1   *Keep a list of the amount and weight of packaging waste that is thrown out from your kitchen in one week. Do you think there is an unnecessary amount? What suggestions can you make to cut down the amount?*

2   *Unpack a packet of biscuits. Comment on the amount of packaging material and how effective it is. Do you think the biscuits were 'overpacked'?*

3   *Think about different ways of designing packages for re-use.*

Recap 6

Complete the following sentences:

1 Harmful bacteria can cause _____.
2 Reheated food must be heated to a _____ temperature.
3 It should be heated _____.
4 Food should be stored in a _____ or a _____.
5 Changing waste into something else is called _____.

Answer the following questions:

6 What conditions do micro-organisms need to multiply?
7 What other conditions affect micro-organisms? Say how.
8 What are 'star ratings'? Explain why they are useful.
9 How can we avoid too much waste in the kitchen? Give as many examples as you can.
10 What causes food spoilage? How can we prevent it?
11 What are the different ways of preserving food? Explain how one of them works.

12 Why do you think it is necessary to wash jam jars carefully when they are empty before you re-use them? Give reasons.

13 Try preserving the following fruit and vegetables in as many ways as you can: Strawberries...cabbage...plums...beans. Which method do you think is the best for each?

7 Food and technology

7.1 Food additives

What are additives?

Additives are substances which are added to food for any of the following reasons:

1 To increase the nutritive value.
2 To improve the cooking qualities of food.
3 To improve the colour, flavour and texture of food.
4 To help food keep better.

The government carefully controls the use of additives in food. The ones which are allowed are called **permitted additives**. You will see them called this on some foods such as sausages.

Types of additives

Monosodium glutamate is a 'flavour intensifier'. It is a salt which increases and blends the flavours of the ingredients. It is found in packet soups, soy sauce and many tinned meals containing meat.

Lecithin is a stabilizer and thickener which prevents mixtures of oil and water from separating e.g. in 'Instant Whip'.

An **anti-splattering agent** is added to cooking fats to stop the fat spitting.

Humectants are added to foods to keep them moist and to stop them becoming stale.

Antioxidants are added to fats and mixtures containing fat to stop them going rancid.

(MSG) Monosodium glutamate	Farina
Meat extract	Sodium nitrate
Hydrolysed protein	Polyphosphates
Yeast extract	Potassium nitrate
Caramel colour	Spirit vinegar
Lactose	Egg
Carageanan	Gum tragacanth
Sodium phosphate	Propylene glycol alginate
Carotenoids	Gelatine
Skimmed milk	Collagen
Buttermilk	Hydrogenated vegetable oil
Partial glycerol estors	Sodium caceinate
Sorbitan tristearate	Propylane glycol monopalmitate
Sodium bisulphite	Lecithin
Butylated hydroxyanisole (BHA)	Sodium citrate
Glyceryl monostearate (GMS)	Citric acid
	Glucose syrup
Non-fat milk solids	Saccharine
Sulphur dioxide	Invert sugar

Tomato soup
Tomatoes, sugar, wheat, salt, edible starch, edible fat, MSG, onion, sodium phosphate, spice and carotenoids.

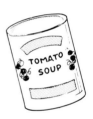

Instant potato
Potatoes, glyceryl, monosteride, non-fat milk solids, sulphur dioxide.

Gravy mix
Farine, salt, caramel, wheat starch, choice vegetable flavourings, yeast, hydrolysed vegetable protein.

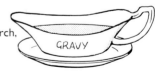

Chopped ham with pork
Ham, pork, spices, polyphosphates, potassium nitrate, sodium nitrate.

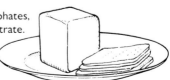

A mystery substance!

Here is a list of ingredients from a packet. Can you guess what is in the packet?

Edible vegetable oil, sugar, permitted emulsifiers, starch, lactose, sodium caseinate, whey powder, lecithin, flavourings, antioxidant, colour.

The packet contains a cream topping which is made up with milk. It can be used in recipes instead of fresh cream. The taste is not the same as fresh cream but there are some advantages in the use of cream topping. These are:

1 It is a powder, and therefore has a long shelf life. This makes it useful for stand-bys and emergencies.
2 The topping is cheaper than the same amount of cream.
3 It contains a smaller proportion of saturated fatty acids than fresh cream.

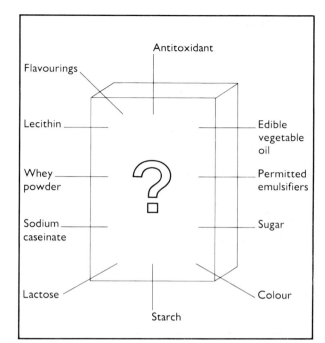

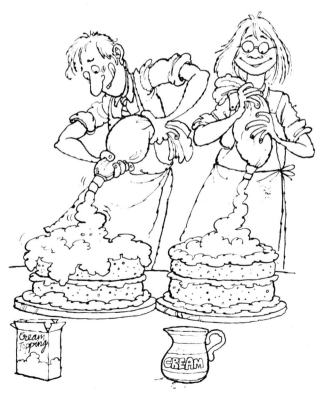

Things to do

1 *Collect the labels from packets and containers and note the additives they have in them. Try to work out why each is there.*

2 *Make a list of foods you have used or eaten that contain nutritional supplements. (Remember that this means they are **fortified**.) Answer the following questions:*
   a *What good is the use of additives in food to the consumer?*
   b *Is the use of additives a controversial subject (one which people disagree about)? If so why?*

3 *Compare the cost of filling and decorating a victoria sandwich with packet cream topping and fresh cream. Compare the time it takes too.*

7.2 Convenience foods

The cream topping in section 7.1 is a good example of a convenience food.

We often think that convenience foods are modern inventions but this is not really true. Self-raising flour and custard powder are convenience foods and these have been available in the shops for a long time.

Why do we use convenience foods?

In the past people used to look for three things when they shopped for food. These were quality, price and convenience, in that order.

Today however, because the shopper is busy and probably working, convenience may come first with quality and cost following. When we buy prepared or partly prepared food we are buying **time**, which we can then use to do something else.

Convenience foods let people prepare a variety of appetizing meals in a very short time. They can raise the standard of family meals. They are also useful for people who cannot cook or who do not like cooking. It is a good idea to keep a few convenience foods stored for use in an emergency. People who live alone or who have poor cooking facilities can make good use of convenience foods to give a wider variety to their diet.

If you use a little imagination you can also use convenience foods in interesting ways. For example, try making up a packet of soup with less liquid than you are told to add and use it as a filling for vegetables such as tomatoes, marrows or onions, as a flavouring in a stew or as a sauce for fish or vegetables.

Boil-in-the-bag foods are very easy to reheat and leave no cooking smells. There is little washing up. This is another advantage of using convenience foods.

Take-away meals are also convenience foods. They are useful when time is short and for emergencies.

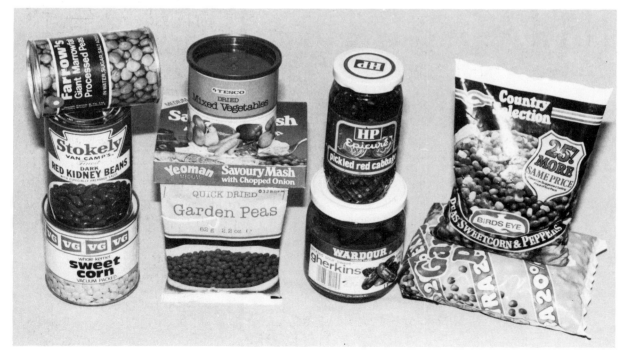

Using convenience foods

When you use convenience foods you should remember the following:

1 A diet which includes too many convenience foods will be **expensive** and **may not be nutritionally sound**.
2 The taste and texture of fresh food is often better than that of the equivalent convenience food.
3 It is wise to eat some fresh food every day, especially fruit and vegetables. A tomato eaten with a take-away hamburger adds the vitamin C which is missing and makes this a nutritious meal when time is short.
4 Convenience foods are best used together with freshly prepared food. An example would be a meat pie made with bought pastry and fresh meat.

You should also watch out for the following:

1 The attractive and tempting way convenience foods are advertised in the shops and on television — this can persuade you to buy things you do not really want.
2 The order of ingredients on packets, cans and food wrappings — the first ingredient in the list is the one the food contains most of, the last is the one the food has the least of. If the meat in a meat product comes near the bottom of the list, there is probably not much meat in the product and its nutritive value may be low. A fruit pie filling which has sugar as its first ingredient does not usually contain a lot of fruit, so it would probably not compare well with another make of fruit pie filling which had fruit as the first ingredient in the list.

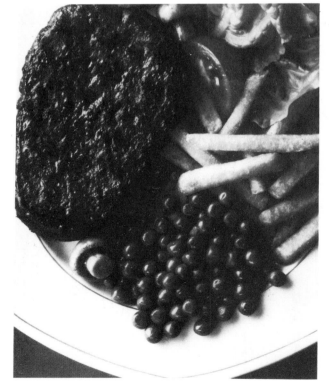

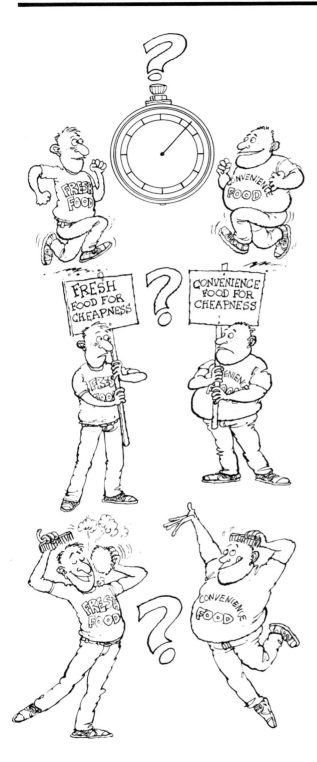

What is the value of convenience foods?

To work out the value of any convenience food you should think about the following:

1 **Time saving** — does it really take less time to use the convenience product than to make a similar dish from fresh ingredients?
2 **Energy and fuel saving** — does the convenience food really involve less preparation and is there any less fuel used to cook it?
3 **Cost** — how does the cost of the convenience food compare with the cost of the fresh food? Remember to include the cost of any extra ingredients you will need to add to the convenience food.
4 **Nutritive value** — this may be difficult to compare sometimes. For example, in the case of 'Instant Whip', the milk used to make it up means that it is just as nutritious as a blancmange.
5 **Appearance** — how does the convenience food compare in colour and texture with the fresh food?
6 **Taste** — is there a big difference between the taste of dishes made from convenience foods and ones made from fresh foods?

Things to do

1 *Compare a packet mix with the corresponding fresh food. Think about all of the things mentioned above. How valuable do you think the convenience food is? Compare your findings with the findings of your friends.*

2 *Draw up a chart to show arguments for and against using convenience foods. Think of as many arguments as you can.*

CONVENIENCE FOOD	
Reasons for	Reasons against

Recap 7

Complete the following sentences:

1 _____ is a flavour intensifier.
2 _____ stop fat from going rancid.
3 Humecants keep foods _____ and stop them going _____.
4 Anti-spattering agents stop _____ from spitting.
5 Lecithin prevents _____.

Are the following statements true or false?

6 Convenience foods are modern inventions.
7 Monosodium glutamate keeps food moist.
8 Convenience foods are usually more expensive than fresh foods.
9 When we buy convenience foods we are buying time.
10 The taste of convenience foods is usually better than fresh foods.

11 Why are additives added to food? Give as many reasons as you can. Explain what 'permitted' additives are.

12 Find out what % of a tin of luncheon meat should be meat. The manager of your local supermarket should be able to help.

13 Make a poster about convenience foods. Draw it out in three columns. Call the first column **Type of food**. List these types of food under the heading:
   a Mixes that need extra ingredients and liquid added.
   b Foods needing short cooking time.
   c Foods needing reconstituting.
   d 'Instant' foods.
   e Foods needing no cooking.
Call the second column **Examples** and put examples of the different types of convenience foods in it. Find pictures of the examples you have given and stick them in the third column.

Revision

Examinations will not frighten you if you work hard during your course and then revise what you have learnt properly. You need to do revision because it is impossible for you to remember everything that you have learnt. You need to remind yourself about all the topics.

If you follow the advice on this page you should be able to enter the examination room confidently and you will be able to tackle the exam more successfully.

When and where to revise

Revise early each evening before you get too tired. Start revising well before exam time.

Do your revision somewhere quiet. For example, your bedroom might be a good place to work. If there is nowhere quiet at home then try working in the reference section of your local library instead.

Make sure that the room is well-lit and not too hot or cold. Work at a table and make sure that you can see a clock as you will need to time yourself carefully (see below).

Planning your revision

Plan your revision carefully. Make sure that you know what the exam syllabus covers. Make sure you revise all the topics.

Revise for a fixed time each day, for example, 2 hours. Split this into short sessions of 25 minutes of revision followed by a short break. This will stop you from getting too tired and your brain will remember things better.

To improve your memory even more, revise the same work again after 10 minutes. You could do this straight after your break. Then revise the work again after 1 day and then once more after 1 week. You will also find you remember things better if you understand them. Ask your teacher about any topic that puzzles you. Make sure that you know and understand the technical words you have learnt.

Testing yourself

Test yourself by doing questions from past exam papers. This will show what you know well and what you need to revise again.

Near the exam time do past exam questions in the time given on the paper. This will get you used to working at the correct speed.

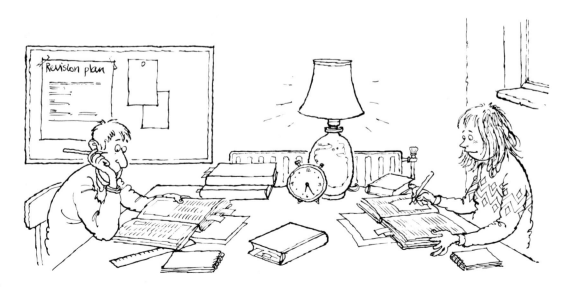

Examinations

Before the exam

Check the date and time of each exam carefully — you don't want to miss the exam after revising so hard!

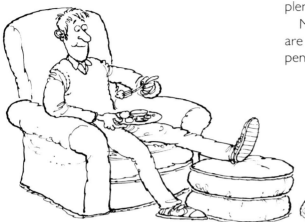

On the day

Do not revise immediately before the exam. Instead relax. *Do* eat before an exam as you will not work well if you are hungry. *Do* allow yourself plenty of time to get to the exam.

Make sure you have everything you need. If you are doing a written exam make sure you have 2 pens, 2 pencils, a rubber a ruler and a watch.

UNITED KINGDOM
EXAMINATIONS BOARD

**CERTIFICATE
OF SECONDARY
EDUCATION**

1985 EXAMINATION

HOME ECONOMICS
PART B: THEORY
TIME ALLOWED: 1½ HOURS

Read the following instructions carefully.

Section A
Answer **all** the Questions 1 to 15.

Section B
Answer **one** question from Questions 1 to 3.

Write your answers in the separate answer book provided.

Note carefully the type of answer required in each section of the paper.

At the end of the examination enter in the column headed 'For Candidate's Use' on the front cover of the answer book the number of the question you have answered from Section B.

The marks allocated to each question are shown on the paper.

In the exam room

First, read the instructions on the front of your paper. Make sure you know how many questions you have to answer. Then work out how much time you should spend on each question.

If you have a choice of questions think carefully about which ones you are going to do.

Obey the instructions in the questions. For example, if a question asks you to list something, don't write long paragraphs about it instead.

Do your best questions first. If you get stuck in the middle of an answer leave a blank and go back later.

If you have to do multiple-choice questions read the instructions very carefully. Make sure you mark your answer opposite the right question number. If you don't know the answer to a question and need to guess, eliminate as many wrong answers as you can. This will improve your chances of getting the answer right.

Above all don't panic! If you have worked well and have revised properly you should have nothing to worry about.

Exam questions

1 a What is a fan-assisted oven?
  b What is the advantage of cooking food in this type of oven compared to an ordinary one?

2 a Name **two** metals which are used for making saucepans.
  b You are about to buy a new saucepan. List **four** points you will look for to ensure that it will be efficient and safe to use.

3 a Explain why a liquid which contains flour thickens when it is heated.
  b What ingredient, other than Quick Jel, could be used to thicken fruit juice which is to be used as a glaze over fruit in a flan?

4 a A date stamp is found on the packaging of some foods. What does the date mean?
  b Name **two** packaged foods which are usually date-stamped.
  c Give **one** reason why date-stamping is a help to the consumer when buying these foods.

5 Make a selection of dishes to show how you would ensure that members of your family had sufficient dietary fibre (roughage) in their meals.

6 a Prepare, cook and display a selection of dishes to store in the freezer. Pack **one** of these dishes for the freezer.
  b Prepare, cook and display a two-course evening meal which would include one of the dishes selected above.

7 a Prepare, cook and serve a breakfast for an old lady living alone. Set either the table or a tray.
  b Prepare, cook and serve a soup which the old lady could have at lunchtime.
  c Prepare, cook and serve a two-course main meal for an elderly couple.

8 State **two** functions of protein in the body.

9 Name the type of protein contained in
  a meat,
  b baked beans.

10 Complete the following sentences:
  a The most important mineral for developing strong bones and teeth is _____.
  b One food which has a good source of this material is _____.

11 Name **two** organisms which cause food spoilage.

12 Name **two** processes by which milk is made safe to drink.

13 Write **four** important points on each of the following:
  a Good hygiene in the kitchen.
  b Pressure cooking.
  c Fuel economy in cooking.

14 Complete the following sentence:
The amount of _____ needed by the body is measured in joules, kilojoules or megajoules.

15 Underline the correct answer.
The multiplication of germs is most rapid when the food is:
  a being thawed.
  b being frozen.
  c kept in a warm kitchen.
  d kept in a larder.
  e kept in a refrigerator.

16 State **four** ways of introducing air into a mixture.

17 a How could each of the following be avoided?
        i Poor teeth
        ii Overweight
        iii Anaemia
    b Is breakfast an important meal? Give reasons for your answer.
    c List the important points to be considered when planning meals for a family.
    d If you were responsible for a school cafeteria, what foods would you offer to encourage children to eat wisely?

18 a Name **two** fat-soluble and **two** water-soluble vitamins and give a good food source of each.
    b Why is a pregnant woman's diet particularly important? Suggest a suitable menu for a two-course meal for her.
    c Give **four** reasons why a person recovering from illness needs a special diet. Give **six** points to remember when preparing and serving food to a person on such a diet.

19 a Give **four** points you would look for in order to decide whether a shop was hygienic.
    b Suggest **six** ways in which the housewife can cut food costs when shopping.
    c Convenience foods are very much part of our national diet today. Give reasons why you think this is so.
       Comment on each of the following aspects of convenience foods:
        i nutritional value,
        ii flavour,
        iii cost.

20 a What is meant by the term 'high biological value' when referring to protein foods? Name **two** good food sources.
    b Give **six** points which should be considered when planning meals.

c Suggest midday meals for the following people and situations, giving reasons for your choice:
    i packed lunch for a teenager at school,
    ii canteen meal for a manual worker.

21 a Name **four** root or tuber vegetables and suggest **four** different ways of using this type of vegetable.
    b When preparing and cooking vegetables, some of the nutrients may easily be destroyed.
       i Which are these nutrients?
       ii Explain fully **four** precautions you can take to ensure the minimum loss of these nutrients.

22 a What are the nutrients found in meat?
    b Give **three** reasons for cooking meat.
    c Name **two** main course dishes using economical cuts of meat.
    d i What is offal?
       ii Give **four** examples of offal.
       iii Name **two** dishes using offal.

23 What is meant by the following?
    a wholemeal flour,
    b self-raising flour,
    c 'strong' or 'hard' flour.

24 In making bread
    a name the **three** conditions necessary for the growth of yeast;
    b name the gas produced to raise the bread;
    c give **two** reasons for kneading the dough;
    d say why it is put in a warm place to rise;
    e give **two** reasons for baking in a hot oven.

25 Give **two** coatings for fish when frying.

26 a From what is pasta made?
    b Name **two** dishes using pasta.

27 a What is TVP?
    b From what is it made?

28 What is meant by the term 'convenience food'?

29 a Name **five** of the most important rules of hygiene to remember when handling and preparing food in the home.
    b What **four** points should be remembered about the storage of food in a refrigerator?
    c State how to store the following items, which were purchased today:
        i fruit cake,
        ii cabbage,
        iii packet of fish fingers,
        iv packet of tea.

30 a What general rules should be followed when planning meals for a person who is ill in bed?
    b Comment on the inclusion of the following nutrients in a convalescent diet:
        i protein,
        ii vitamins,
        iii minerals.
    c The meal below is a suggested menu for a convalescent. Give **one** reason why each of the dishes is suitable to be included in the meal.

        Chicken casserole
        Carrots
        Spinach
        Creamed potatoes
        Chocolate mousse
        Shortbread fingers
        Homemade lemonade

31 a Explain how food is cooked in a microwave oven.
    b What care is needed to ensure the efficient use of a microwave oven?

32 a What are the causes of decay in fruit and vegetables?
    b What are the principles underlying the preservation of fruit and vegetables? Explain how these principles are applied in the various methods of preservation of fruit and vegetables.
    c Explain in detail how you would preserve **two** of the following:
        i rhubarb by bottling,
        ii raspberries by making jam,
        iii onions by pickling.

33 a Write an informative paragraph about the protein found in cows' milk.
    b List the other nutrients which are found in cows' milk.
    c What is skimmed milk? State the nutritional advantages and disadvantages of using this type of milk.

34 a Discuss the advantages and disadvantages of buying and using the commercially prepared foods on sale in the shops. Describe the role they should play in the preparation of meals.
    b Why is it important to read the labels on packets and tins of food?
    c The following substances are frequently found in convenience foods. For each one, suggest one reason for its inclusion in the product:
        i monosodium glutamate,
        ii anti-oxidant,
        iii emulsifier,
        iv colouring.

Careers

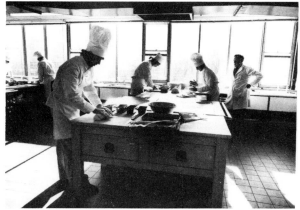

Learning how to be a chef

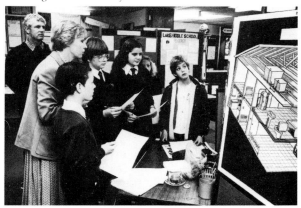

Teaching

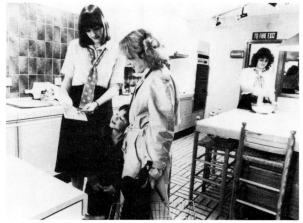

Public relations

Have you decided what you want to do when you leave school?

You will find home economics qualifications particularly useful for these types of work:
Catering
Equipment testing and development
Food technology
Hotel training
Marketing
Nursery nursing
Nursing
Public relations
Recipe testing and development
Social services
Teaching

For many of these you will need to study further at school, at a 6th Form college or in a college of further education. Your careers teacher should be able to give you more details of this.

There are also three books published by the Careers Research and Advisory Committee (CRAC) which you can read. They are called:

Decisions at 13/14
Decisions at 15/16
Your choice at 17+

You can get them from CRAC at Bateman Street, Cambridge.

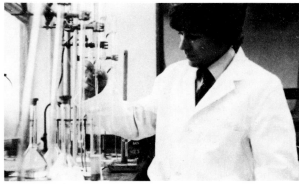

Food technology

Index

A
Air 78
Aluminium 90
Amino acids 7, 8
Anaemia 37
Antioxidants 108
Antisplattering agents 108
Aseptic canning 101

B
Bacteria 44, 60, 94, 95-107
Baking powder 79
Bicarbonate of soda 78
Binding (egg) 58
Boil in the bag 110
Borosilicate 92
Bran 69
Breakfast 27
Bromelin 51

C
Calcium carbonate 56
Calcium 19, 53
Canteen meals 29
Carbon dioxide 78-9, 82-3
Casein 60
Cast iron 91
Cellulose 45
Chicken 50
Cholesterol 45
Chute 106
Clostridium botulinus 94
Clostridium welchii 94
Collagen 51, 54
Complementation 8
Condensed milk 62
Conduction 84
Connective tissue 51, 54
Convection 84
Crustaceans 54
Custard powder 110

D
Dextrin 76
Diabetes 42
Dietary fibre 5
Durum wheat 71

E
Earthenware 92
Elastin 51
Endosperm 69
Energy conservation 30
Enzyme action 97
Evaporated milk 62
Extending proteins 9
Extraction 70

F
Fats and oils (lipids) 5, 11
Fatty acids 11
Fermentation 79, 82-3
Fibre 5
Fluoridation 21
Fluorine 19, 21, 53

Fortification 9
Fuel 25

G
Gall bladder disease 42
Gelatin 51
Gelatinization 72
Germ 69
Gliadin 80
Glucose 12
Glutenin 80
Glutin 80
Glycerol 11
Grain 69

H
Haemoglobin 19
Hay box 88
High temperature short term canning
   101
Higher biological value protein 7
Humectants 108
Hydrogen sulphide 57

I
Infective food poisoning 94
Inhibitors 37
Invisible fat 11

J
Junket 60

K
Kilojoule 13

L
Lactic acid 60
Lecithin 58, 108
Low fat food 47, 62-3
Lower biological value protein 7

M
Magneton 86
Main meals 30
Marinade 51-2
Mayonnaise 58
Micro-organisms 95-107
Microwave cooker 30, 86
Midday meal 28, 29
Minerals 5, 18
Molluscs 54
Monosodium glutamate 108
Moulds 97
Myosin 51

N
Non-stick coatings 91
Nutrition 6
Nutritional supplements 37

O
Obesity 42
Offal 50
Oils 5, 11
Oxidase 77

Oxidation 12

P
Papain 51
Phosphorus 56
Phytic acid 37
Potassium 19
Pressure cooking 25, 30, 75
Protein 5
Proteolytic enzymes 51
Pyroceram 90

R
Rabbit 50
Radiation 84, 85
Recommended amounts of nutrients 8
Recycling waste 106
Refrigeration 103
Riboflavin 56

S
Salmonella 94
Saturated fatty acids 45
Self-raising flour 110
Sell by date 31
Shops 31-5
Slow cooking 88-9
Sodium 19, 21
Staphylococci 94
Staple foods 70-1
Starch 5, 10
Star ratings 104, 107
Sublimation 98
Sugars 5, 10
Sulphur dioxide 99

T
Textured vegetable protein 9
Thyroxine 19
Thiamin 56

U
Unit price 31
Unsaturated fatty acids 45

V
Visible fat 11
Vitamin A 15, 53, 56, 60
Vitamin B 16
Vitamin C 6, 17, 38, 66, 67, 68, 77
Vitamin D 16, 53, 56
Vitamins 5, 14, 15

W
Waste disposal units 106
Weak flour 80
Whole foods 46
Wholemeal flour 70

Y
Yeast 78, 79, 82, 83

Z
Zoned heat 87